Kamilia Laabadi

Clinical, radiological and histological correlation of breast tumors

Kamilia Laabadi

Clinical, radiological and histological correlation of breast tumors

About 250 cases

ScienciaScripts

Imprint

Any brand names and product names mentioned in this book are subject to trademark, brand or patent protection and are trademarks or registered trademarks of their respective holders. The use of brand names, product names, common names, trade names, product descriptions etc. even without a particular marking in this work is in no way to be construed to mean that such names may be regarded as unrestricted in respect of trademark and brand protection legislation and could thus be used by anyone.

Cover image: www.ingimage.com

This book is a translation from the original published under ISBN 978-613-8-45550-9.

Publisher:
Sciencia Scripts
is a trademark of
Dodo Books Indian Ocean Ltd. and OmniScriptum S.R.L publishing group

120 High Road, East Finchley, London, N2 9ED, United Kingdom
Str. Armeneasca 28/1, office 1, Chisinau MD-2012, Republic of Moldova, Europe
Managing Directors: Ieva Konstantinova, Victoria Ursu
info@omniscriptum.com

Printed at: see last page
ISBN: 978-620-4-04600-6

Table of contents:

Clinical, radiological and histological correlation of palpable breast tumours (about 250 cases)

Introduction:

Tumor pathology of the breast is extremely common, with 8 to 9 out of 10 women coming to the clinic with a breast problem (1, 2, 3). Although less common than benign mastopathy, breast cancer is the most common tumor in women and is the leading cause of cancer death in women, making it a real public health problem.

The management of a breast nodule involves following a well-defined diagnostic procedure.

The clinical examination has been for centuries and still is today at the forefront of this approach. However, when a suspicious mass is palpated, the diagnosis is often delayed and a normal clinical examination does not rule out cancer; hence the interest in mammographic screening. Mammography is a reliable and non-invasive technique that has proven its effectiveness in the field of screening.

Currently, with the rejuvenation of the population, breasts are denser, which affects the sensitivity of mammography and gives even more importance to ultrasound in the diagnosis of breast tumors.

Percutaneous sampling of breast lesions is increasingly common. For a long time, they were limited to an easy and less expensive cytopunction allowing cellular analysis of the lesion, but leading to a certain number of false negatives or non-contributing samples. For a long time, this examination was requested as a first-line procedure, but it has now been abandoned in view of the possibility of taking histological samples (micro- or macro-biopsy) which allow histological analysis of tissue fragments.

Through this retrospective study, from January 2011 to December 2012 about 250 cases of breast tumors collected in the department of obstetrics gynecology II of Hassan II University Hospital of FES; we will specify the respective values of clinical, mammography, ultrasound and confront them with the definitive anatomical-pathological examination to study the sensitivity and specificity of each method.

I. Materials and Methods

Our work consists of a retrospective study of a series of 250 patients collected in the department of gyneco-obstetrics II at the Hassan II University Hospital of Fez during 2 years (2011-2012).

This work was carried out through a consultation of the patients' files in the archives.

Inclusion criteria

All women with breast lesion(s) who had ultrasound and mammography with histological evidence of the breast lesion were included.

Non-inclusion criteria

We excluded from this study, the sub-clinical lesions of the breast **Statistical exploitation and analysis of the results :**

The results are presented in tabular form, analyzed descriptively and correlationally.

For the realization of this work, we have consulted :

- Clinical data.

- Imaging results.

- Anatomopathological reports.

For each patient, we noted:

< Age

< Background

< Hormonal status

< Management and parity

< Reason for consultation

< Clinical examination

< Mammogram results

< The results of the breast ultrasound

< histological findings

II. Results

1. EPIDEMIOLOGICAL PROFILE :

A– <u>Age of discovery</u> :

The age of our patients ranged from 17 to 78 years with an average of 47.5 years.
The age group most affected is 26-45 years, representing 38.4% of the cases in our
sample

Table 1: Distribution of patients by 10-year age group

Age (years)	Number of cases	Percentage (%)
15-25	51	20,4
26-35	36	14,4
36-45	60	24
46-55	53	21,2
56 years and over	50	20
Total	250	100

The most represented age group was between 36 and 45 years old, followed by
those between 26 and 35 years old.

Figure 1: Distribution of patients by 10-year age group

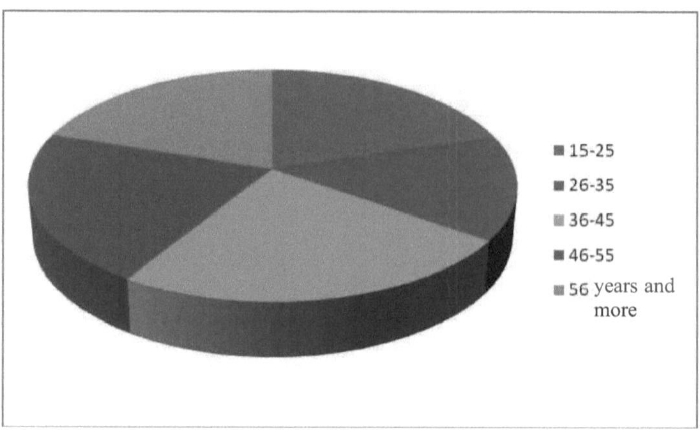

8- <u>Background</u>:

1- Staff :

6 patients had a history of contralateral breast cancer, i.e. 2.4% of cases.
A history of benign mastopathy was found in 9 patients, i.e. 3.6% of cases.
One patient had a history of Krukenberg's tumor
One patient had a history of sigmoidal cancer

2- Family :

The search for breast cancer revealed 6 cases, 3 in the sister, 1 in the mother and 1 in the maternal aunt.

C- <u>PARITY :</u>

Table 2: Distribution of patients by parity

Parity	Number of cases	Percentage (%)
Nulliparous	66	26,4
Pauciparous <2	81	32,4
Multiparous >3	103	41,2

Multiparity was noted in 41.2% of all cases, followed by pauci parity, while the number of nulliparous women came last with a percentage of 26.4%.

Figure 2: Distribution of patients by parity

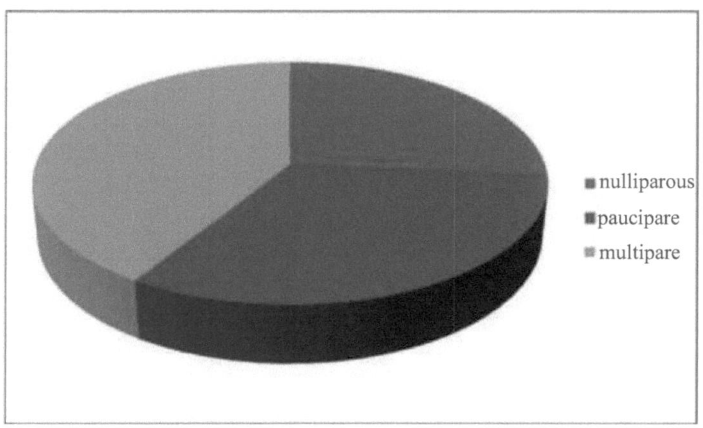

D- <u>Age of puberty :</u>

Table 3: Distribution by age of puberty

Age of puberty	Number of cases	Percentage (%)
10	4	1,6
11	8	3,2
12	60	24
13	71	28,4
14	89	35,6
15	6	2,4
16	10	4
NP	2	0,8
total	250	100

The age of puberty ranged from 10 to 16 years with an average of 14 years. Only 3.2% of patients had their first menstrual period at age 11, compared to 35.6% at age 14.

E- <u>Hormonal status:</u>

Table 4: Distribution by hormonal status

Hormonal status	Number of cases	Percentage (%)
Genital activity	167	66,8
Menopause	83	33,2
Total	250	100

In our series, 167 cases, i.e. 66.8% of the patients were in the genital activity period.
The age of menopause ranged from 47 to 54 years with a mean of 50.5 years.
The late menopause rate is 53.7% of menopausal women. Graph 3: Distribution according to hormonal status

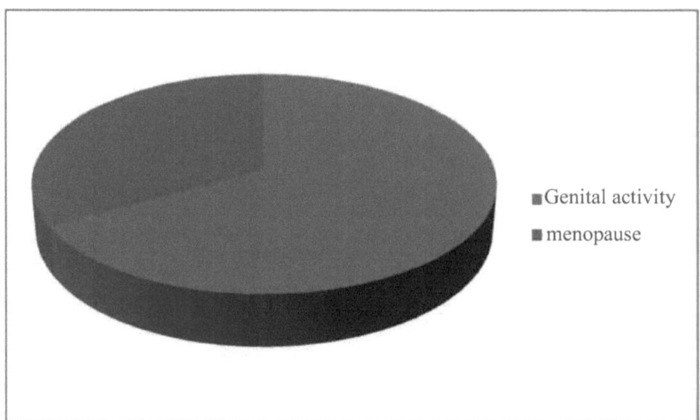

F- <u>Age of first pregnancy :</u>

Table 5: Distribution by age at first pregnancy :

Age of first pregnancy (years)	Number of cases	Percentage (%)
<15 years	4	1,6
15–19	26	10,4
20–25	102	40,8
26–30	67	26,8
>30 years	51	20,4
Total	250	100

The maximum frequency is between the ages of 20 and 25; that is, 55% of cases.

Figure 4: Distribution by age of first pregnancy

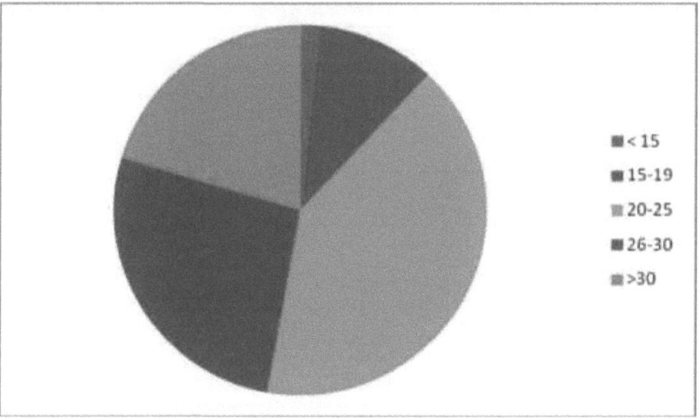

G– Breastfeeding :

Breastfeeding was noted in 178 patients, i.e. 71.2% of cases.

Formula feeding in 6 patients.

66 patients did not breastfeed because they were nulliparous.

H– Taking oral contraceptives :

This parameter was sought in all patients, 140 of whom had taken oral contraceptives, i.e. 56% of the cases. The type of pill could not be specified in 127 cases, whereas it was of the oestroprogestogenic type in 57 cases.

An average duration of exposure to hormonal contraceptives of 6.7 years.

<u>**I– Hormone replacement therapy :**</u>

None of our patients had undergone hormone replacement therapy.

2. CLINICAL DATA

A– <u>Circumstances of discovery :</u>

Table 6: Distribution of patients by reason for consultation :

Reason for consultation	Workforce	Percentage (%)
tumefaction	242	96,8
Mastodynia	1	0,4
Mammalian flow	2	0,8
Skin signs	5	2
Axillary ADP	0	0
total	250	100

Breast nodule was the most frequent reason for consultation with 96.8% of all cases followed by mastodynia with only 0.4%.

Figure 4: Distribution of patients by reason for consultation

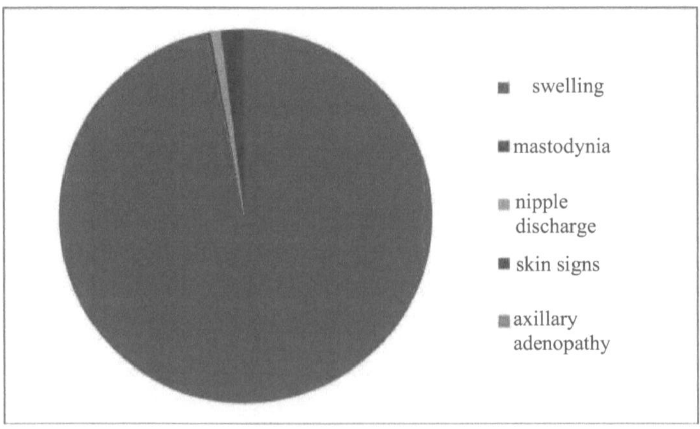

Table 7: Distribution of patients according to the time elapsed between the discovery of the lesion and the consultation

Duration (months)	Workforce	Percentage (%)
0–6 months	88	35,2
6–12 months	124	49,6
>12 months	38	15,2
Total	250	100

49.6% of the patients took between 6 and 12 months to consult the doctor after discovering the breast lesion, against only 15.2% of the cases who remained without consultation beyond 12 months.

Graph 6: Distribution of patients according to the time elapsed between the discovery of the lesion and the consultation

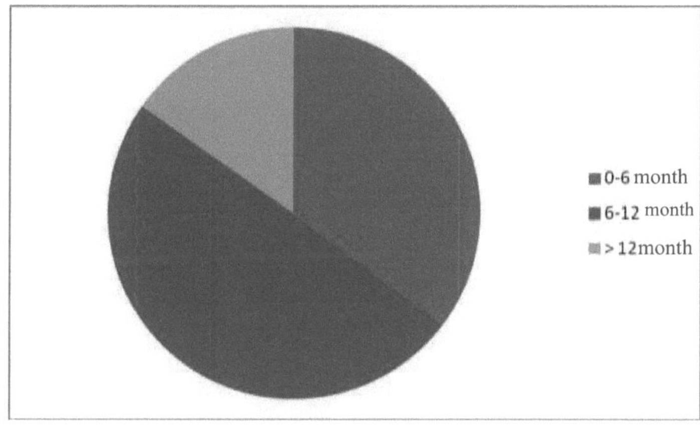

B-Clinical examination :

1) Inspection :

Asymmetry of the two breasts was found in 71 patients, i.e. 28.4%; of which 59 cases of invasive cancer, 12 benign masthopathies and 6 intermediate tumours.
Mammary retraction was found in 34 patients, 30 of whom (88.3%) had a histological diagnosis of invasive cancer, with only 4 cases of intermediate tumours (11.7%).
The orange peel was observed in 28 patients whose histological diagnosis was in favour of malignancy in all cases.
Redness was seen in 18 patients (7.2%). Curvature was seen in 69 patients (27.6%).

2) Palpation:
a) Number of lesions:

Table 8: Distribution of patients according to the number of swellings on clinical examination :

Number of palpable nodules	Workforce	Percentage (%)
1	213	85,2
2 à 3	34	13,6
> à 3	3	1,2
Total	250	100

In 85.2% of cases, the lesion was unique (213 patients). Gra

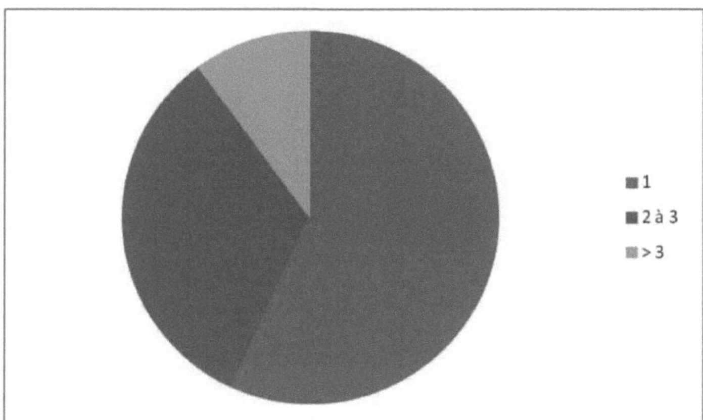

b) Size:

Size (cm)	No. Malignant tumor	Number of benign tumours	No. of intermediate tumors	total	Percentage (%)
<2	19	29	7	55	22
2<−< 5	95	45	13	153	61,2
5<−< 10	21	7	0	28	11,2
>10	1 1	3	0	14	5,6
total	146	84	20	250	100

Table 9: Distribution by tumour size

The tumor was diagnosed at a size between 2 and 5 cm in 61.2% of cases.

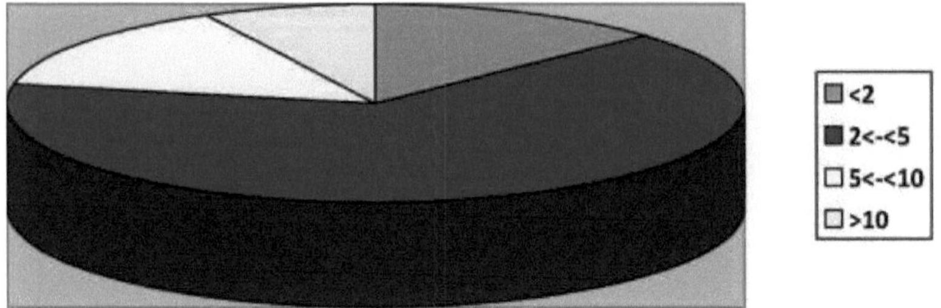

Figure 6: Table 9: Distribution by tumor size

(c) Seat:

There is a slight predominance of tumor location in the left breast (52.7%).
The upper-external quadrant was the most frequent tumor location with a rate of 37%.
The tumor was bilateral in 8 patients or 5.36% of cases.

TNM classification :

- T: tumor size :

22% of patients are classified as T2 (between 2 and 5 cm)
5.6% of our patients were classified as T4 (tumours with extension to the wall and/or skin and inflammatory tumours).

T	Number of cases	percentage
T1	55	22
T2	153	61,2
T3	28	11,2
T4	14	5,6
total	250	100

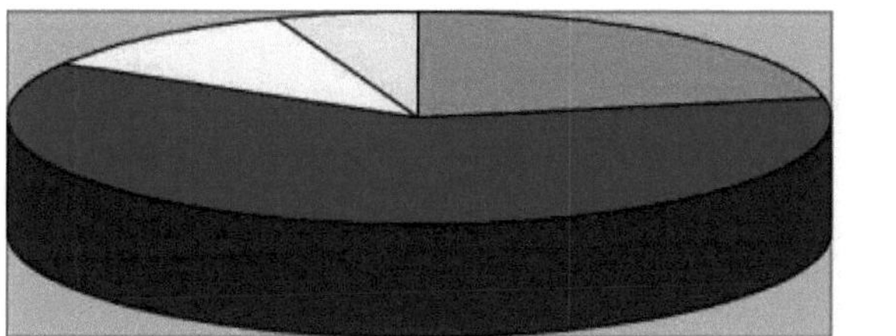

Figure 7: Distribution by tumour stage

Headquarters	Workforce	Percentage (%)
External Super Quadrant	90	36
Internal supero quadrant	26	10,4
External infero quadrant	24	9,6
Internal infero quadrant	12	4,8
Areolar Retro	37	14,8
The whole breast	2	0,8
Axillary extension	9	3,6
Upper quadrant junction	28	11,2
Junction lower quadrants	7	2,8
Int. quadrant junction	3	1,2
Ext. quadrant junction	9	3,6
Inframammary fold	3	1,2
Total	250	100

Table 10: Distribution by tumour location

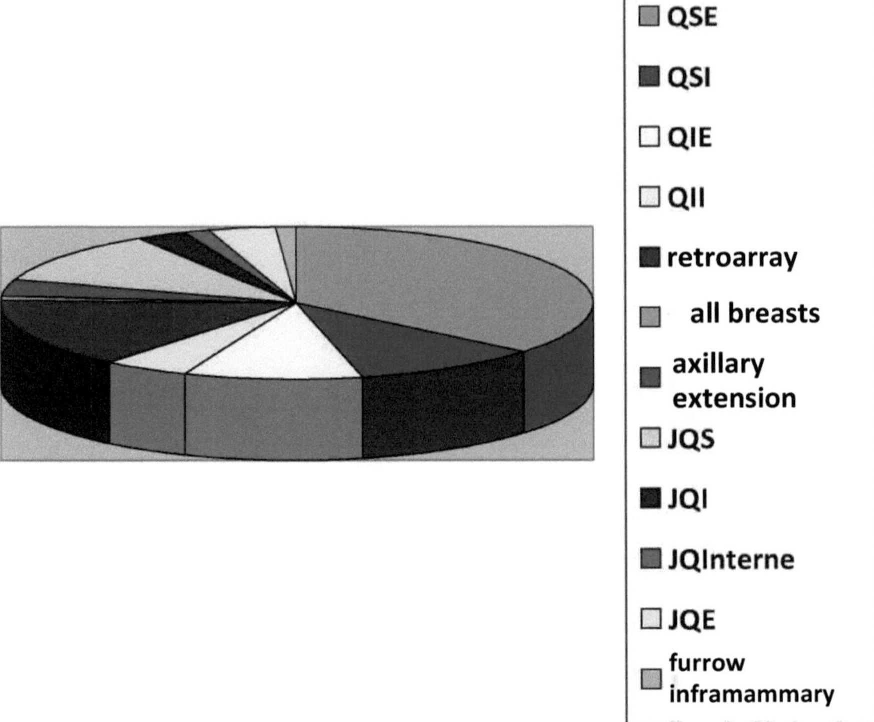

Graph 8: Distribution according to tumour location

(d) Form :

Form	Number of cases			total	Percentage (%)
	Malignant tumours	Benign tumours	Intermediate tumors		
Round	7	49	13	69	27,6
oval	12	26	3	41	16,4

irregular	127	9	4	140	56
total	146	84	20	250	100

Table 11: Distribution of patients according to the shape of the palpable nodule

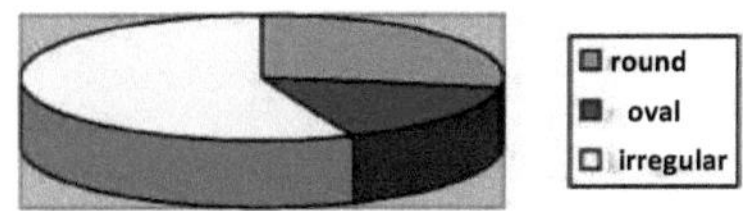

Figure 9: Distribution of patients according to the shape of the palpable nodule

e) Outline :

Table 12: Distribution of patients according to the contours of palpable nodules

forms	Number of cases			total	Percentage (%)
	Malignant tumours	Benign tumours	Intermediate tumors		
Well limited	20	69	3	92	36 ,8
Ill–limited	126	15	17	158	63,2
total	146	84	20	250	100%

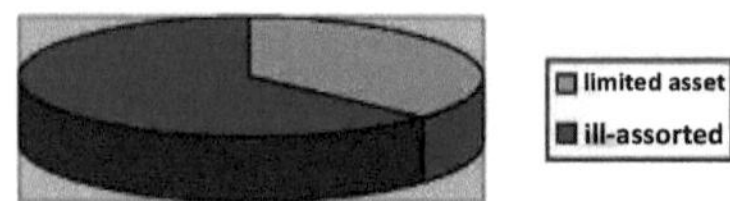

Figure 10: Distribution of patients according to the contours of palpable nodules

Nodules were well limited in 36.8% of cases, of which benign tumours accounted for 75%.
They were poorly limited in 63.2% of cases, of which malignant tumours accounted for 79.7%.

f) mobility and consistency :

Mobility	Workforce	Percentage (%)
Mobile in relation to the 2 planes	180	72%
Mobile/deep plane– fixed/surface plane	6	2,4%
Fixed/deep plane/mobile/surface plane	57	22,8%
Fixed/deep plane – fixed/surface plane	7	2,8%
Total	250	100

Table 13: Distribution of palpable tumours by mobility

72% of the nodules palpable on clinical examination were mobile against only 28% that were adherent.

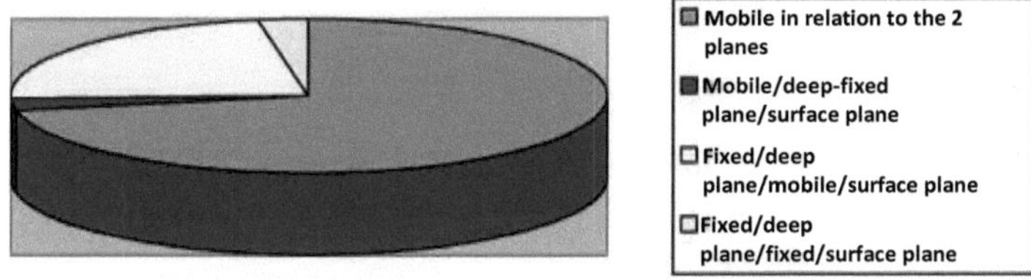

Figure 11: Distribution of palpable tumours by mobility

Consistency	Workforce	Percentage (%)
Farm	146	58,4%
hard	99	39,6%
soft	5	2%
total	250	100

Table 14: Distribution of palpable tumours by consistency

58.4% of the nodules were firm and 39.6% were hard, while soft consistency represented only 2%.

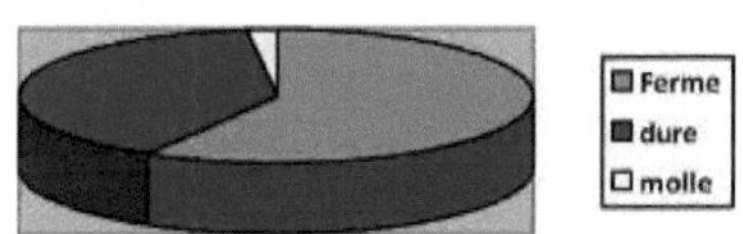

Figure 12: Distribution of palpable tumours by consistency

g) Mammelon flow :

Nipple discharge was found in 2 patients associated with other clinical signs. It was bloody multiporous in one case and serous uniporic in one case.

3) Evolutionary thrust:

88.4% of patients had EPI0 breast cancer.
29 patients had inflammatory breast cancer, of which 6 cases had a progressive EPI3 flare.
No inflammatory manifestations were observed in benign tumors.

EPI stage	number of cases	Percentage (%)
PEV0	221	88,4%
PEV1	8	3,2%
PEV2	10	4%
EPI3	6	2,4%
NP	5	2%
total	250	100

Table 15: Breakdown by growth stage

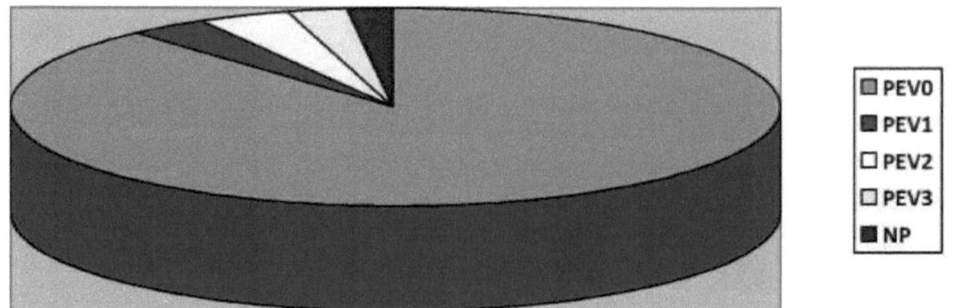

Graph 14: Distribution according to the evolutionary thrust

4) Lymph node involvement:

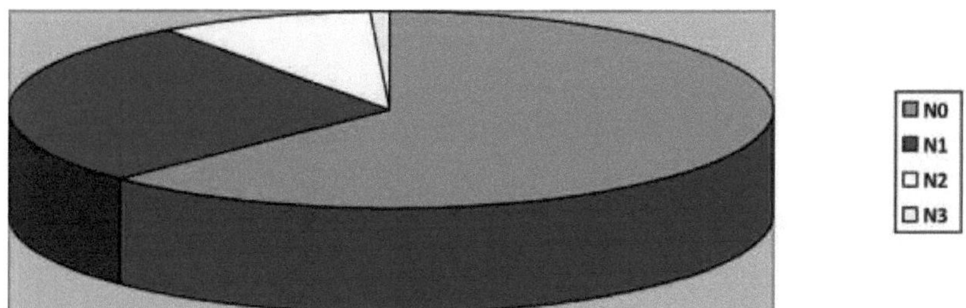

Lymph node	Number of cases	Percentage (%)
N0	156	62,4%
N1	69	27,6%
N2	23	9,2%
N3	2	0,8%
Total	250	100%

Table 16: Distribution according to lymph node involvement

Figure 15: Distribution according to lymph node involvement

38% of the patients had homo, contralateral or supra clavicular or internal mammary adenopathies

5) presence of metastasis :

Table 17: presence or absence of metastasis at the time of consultation

Presence of metastasis	Number of cases	Percentage (%)
MO	234	93,6%
M1	16	6,4%
total	250	100

Table 17: Presence or absence of metastasis at the time of consultation 93.6% of patients were non-metastatic.

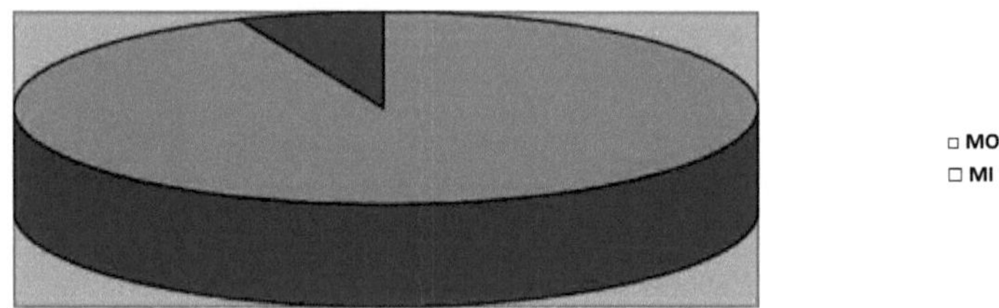

Figure 16: Presence or absence of metastasis at the time of consultation

6) Clinical conclusion:

Among the 250 patients in our study:
In 80 cases were clinically benign, i.e. 32% of cases,
In 123 cases were clinically malignant, i.e. 49.2% of the cases, and only in 47 cases the clinic was inconclusive, i.e. 18.8% of the cases.

1. Radiological data:

Para-clinical	Number of cases	Percentage (%)
Mammography	213	85,2
Ultrasound	250	100

Table 18: Para-clinical examinations

All our patients had a breast ultrasound, while only 85.2% had a mammogram. In the other cases, mammography could not be performed because of the young age (very dense breast) or because of the inflammatory nature of the breast.

A. <u>Mammography</u> :

1. Mammographic aspects encountered :

Opacity was found in 198 patients, or 79.2% of cases.

It was isolated in 152 patients (61%), and associated with microcalcifications in 46 patients.

Mammography was inconclusive, showing very dense breasts in 28 patients, or 11% of cases.

<u>It returned normal in 3 cases of benign masthopathy.</u>

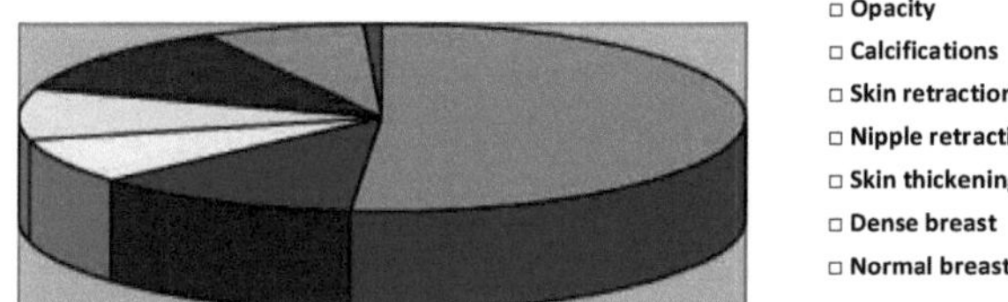

Results	Workforce	Percentage (%)
Opacity	198	79,2%
Calcifications	46	18,4%
Skin shrinkage	30	12%
Nipple retraction	34	13,6%
Skin thickening	46	18,4%
Dense breast	28	11,2%
Normal breast	3	1,2%

Table 19: Mammographic aspects encountered

Graph 17: Mammographic aspects encountered

2. Tumor size on mammography :

Size (cm)	Number of cases	Percentage (%)
< 2	25	10%
2< – <5	135	54%
5< – <10	50	20%
>10	3	1,2%
Total	250	100%

Table 20: Distribution by tumour size
Most breast tumours were between 2 and 5 cm in mammographic size, accounting for 54% of cases.

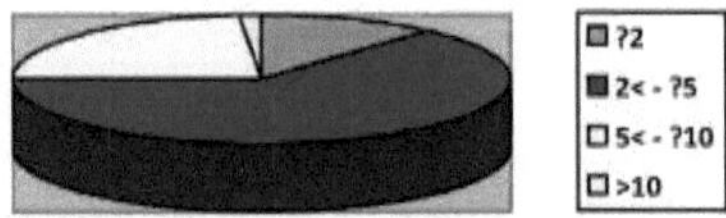

Figure 18: Distribution by tumour size

3- Criteria for benign tumors :

Out of 84 cases of benign tumors, mammography objectified:
– 18 patients presented with dense breasts that could not be explored by mammography, i.e.
21.4% of all benign tumours.
• 57 patients had opacities

• Micro calcifications in 4 cases (4.7%)

• 4 cases of density asymmetry of which 3 cases are associated with other mammographic signs and only 1 case is isolated.
• Mammography returned normal (ACR1) in 3 cases.

> **Opacity :**

Table 21: Distribution by opacity characteristics :

Opacity characteristics		Number of cases	Percentage (%)
Form	–round	33	57,8
	–ovale	18	31,6
	–lobulated	2	3,5
	–irregular	4	7
Number	–1	38	66,7
	–2	11	19,2
	-> 3	8	14,1
Contours	–circumcised	49	86
	–indistincts	2	3,5
	–spiculated	2	3,5
	micro lobules	3	5,2
	–masked	1	1,8
Density	– strong	12	21
	–average	29	51
	–low	8	14
	–greaser	8	14

Well circumscribed opacity was found in 86% of cases.

Spiculated and micro lobulated opacity presented in only 8.7% of cases.

Rounded and oval opacity was found in 89.4% of cases.

"Micro calcifications :

2 cases of micro-calcifications were classified as ACR3 one was classified as ACR2 and one as ACR4

<u>**"Glandular architecture:**</u>
It was modified in one case of benign mastopathy, representing 3.5% of cases.

<u>**"Skin coating :**</u>
Mammography showed skin thickening in front of the tumor in three cases (5.26%).

<u>**"Seat:**</u>
The most frequent site of benign tumors was the upper external quadrant, presenting 50.8% of cases (29 cases).
The second most common location was the retroareolar site (17.5%).

Headquarters	Number of cases	Percentage (%)
Upper outer quadrant	43	52%
Superior Internal Quadrant	6	7,1%
Lower outer quadrant	4	4,8%
Innermost quadrant	4	4,8%
Areolar Retro	15	17,8%
Upper quadrant junction	4	4,8%
Junction lower quadrants	2	2,8%
Int. quadrant junction	3	3,5%
Ext. quadrant junction	3	3,5%
total	84	100%

Table 22: Distribution of benign tumours by site

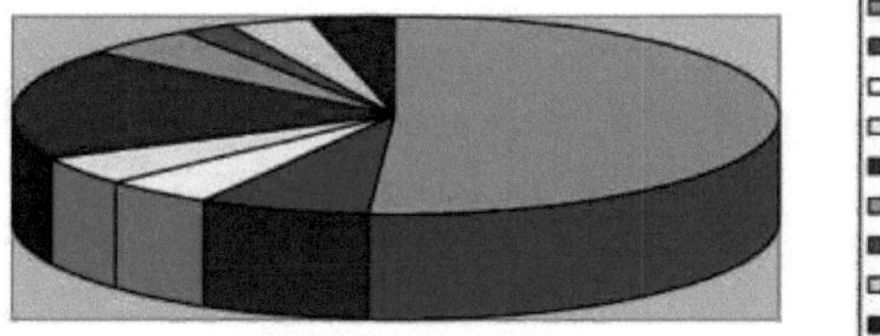

Figure 19: Distribution of benign tumours by site

4) Criteria for malignancy :

> **Opacity :**

Opacity characteristics		Number of cases	Percentage (%)
Form	–round	12	8,5
	–ovale	10	7,1
	–lobulated	27	19,2
	–irregular	92	65,2
Number	–1	121	85,8
	–2	1 5	10,6
	-> 3	5	3,6
Contours	–circumcised	3	2,1
	–indistincts	51	36,2
	–spiculated	78	55,3
	micro lobules	8	5,7
	overcapacity	1	0,7
Density	– strong	23	16,3
	–average	59	41,8
	–low	45	31,9
	–greaser	1 5	10,6

Table 23: Distribution by type of opacity

Of the 146 malignant tumours, opacity was found in 141 patients, i.e. 96.6% of cases.

The most frequent form was opacity with irregular boundaries, with an average of 65.2% of cases.

Spicules were found in 78 patients, i.e. 55.3% of cases.

Additional opacity was found in only 1 patient, i.e. 0.7% of cases.

"Micro calcifications :

They were found in 38 cases, i.e. 26%.

Type of micro calcifications	Number of cases	Percentage (%)
ACR3	4	10 ,5
ACR4	13	34,2
ACR5	21	55,3

Table 24: Type of micro calcifications according to ACR classification.

In our series, the majority of microcalcifications were classified as ACR5 with an average of 55.3% of all microcalcifications.

Microcalcifications classified as ACR4 were second with an average of 34.2%.

Microcalcifications classified as ACR3 were found in 10.5% of cases.

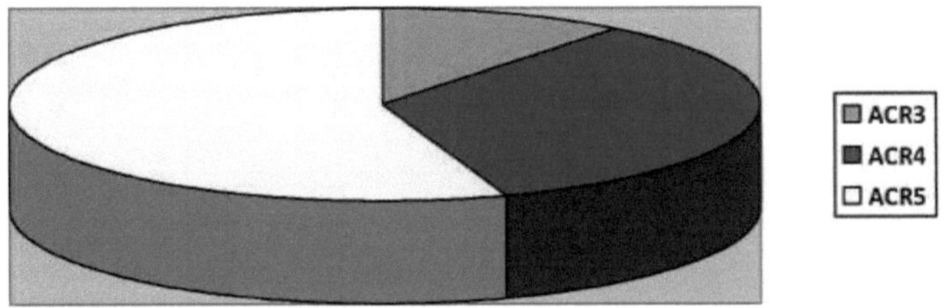

Figure 21: Type of micro calcifications according to ACR classification.

<u>**Associated signs :**</u>

Skin thickening was found in 43 patients, i.e. 17.2% of cases.

Skin retraction was present in 30 cases (17.2%).

Nipple retraction was observed in 34 patients, i.e. 13.6% of cases.

> **Headquarters:**

Headquarters	Number of cases	Percentage (%)
External Super Quadrant	71	48,6%
Internal supero quadrant	25	17,1%
External infero quadrant	8	5,7%
Internal infero quadrant	4	2,7%
Areolar Retro	14	9,6%
Axillary extension	6	4,1%
Upper quadrant junction	11	7,5%
Junction lower quadrants	2	1,3%
Ext. quadrant junction	5	3,4%

Table 25: Distribution of malignant tumours by site

The superolateral quadrant was the most frequent site, representing 48.6% of cases, followed by the superomedial quadrant with 17.1% of cases

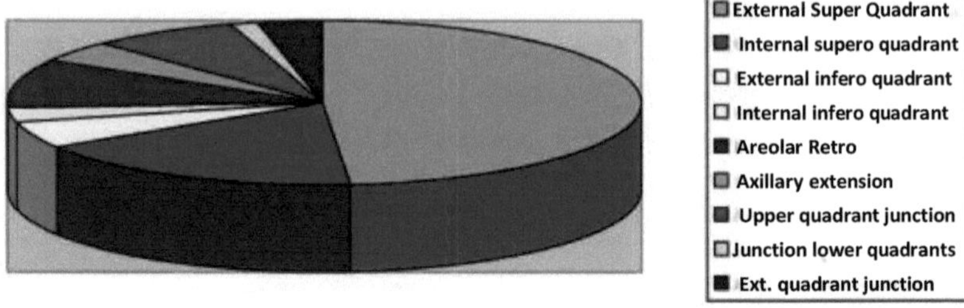

Figure 21: Distribution of malignant tumours by site

5) **intermediate tumors** :

Intermediate tumours presented on mammography as rounded opacities in 4 cases, oval in 7 cases, well circumscribed in 7 cases and indistinct in 2 cases, associated with microcalcifications classified as ACR 3 in 4 cases
The most frequent site was the supero external quadrant found in 13 patients.

6) **Mammographic diagnosis:**

Table 26: Mammographic Diagnosis

Diagnosis	Number of cases	percentage
ACR1	2	0,8%
ACR2	14	5,6%
ACR3	38	15,2%
ACR4	61	24,4%
ACR5	86	34,4%
Inconclusive	12	4,8%
Not done	37	14,8%
Total	250	100%

Table 26: Mammographic Diagnosis

Mammography was normal (ACR1) in two cases 0.8% of cases.
It showed the existence of a benign anomaly (ACR2) in 14 cases, i.e.

5.6% of cases.

Mammographic abnormalities were probably benign (ACR3) in 38 patients or 15.2% of cases.

61 patients had abnormalities suspicious for malignancy (ACR4), representing 24.4% of cases.

Mammography evoked cancer (ACR5) in 86 patients, i.e. 34.4% of cases.

It was inconclusive in 12 patients.

It could not be performed in 14.8% of cases due to the young age of the patients or the inflammatory nature of the breasts.

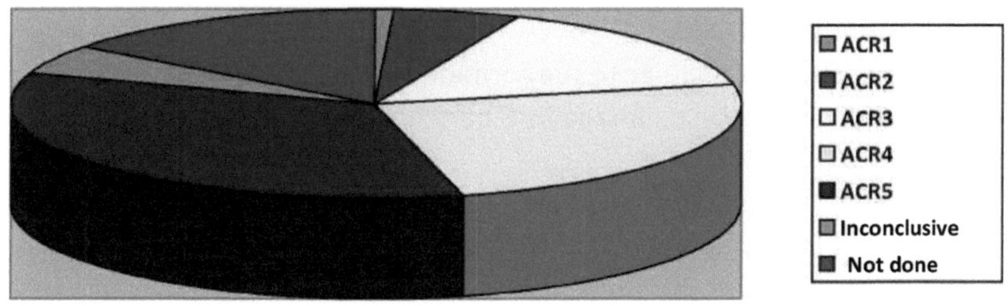

Table 26: Mammographic Diagnosis

B. Ultrasound :

It was the second most frequently requested test.

1) Ultrasound aspects encountered :

Ultrasound data	Number of cases	percentage
Nodular image	242	96,8
Cystic image	8	3,2
Axillary adenopathy	128	51,12
Infiltration of neighbouring tissues	78	31,2
Dilatations of the galactophore ducts	6	2,4
Calcifications	19	7,6

Table 27: Ultrasound Data

242 patients showed nodular tissue formations on ultrasound, i.e. 96.8% of cases.

Ultrasound showed a cystic image in 8 patients, i.e. 3.2% of the
case

Axillary adenopathy was observed in 128 patients or 51.12% of cases.

Dilatation of the galactophore ducts was found in 6 patients, i.e.
2.4% of cases.

Calcifications in 19 patients or 7.6% of cases.

2): Tumor size on ultrasound

Size (cm)	Number of cases	Percentage (%)
< 2	58	23,2%
2< – <5	158	63,2%
5< – <10	27	10,8%
>10	7	2,8%

Table 27: Size distribution.

The tumor size varies between 2 and 5 cm in 63.2% of cases.

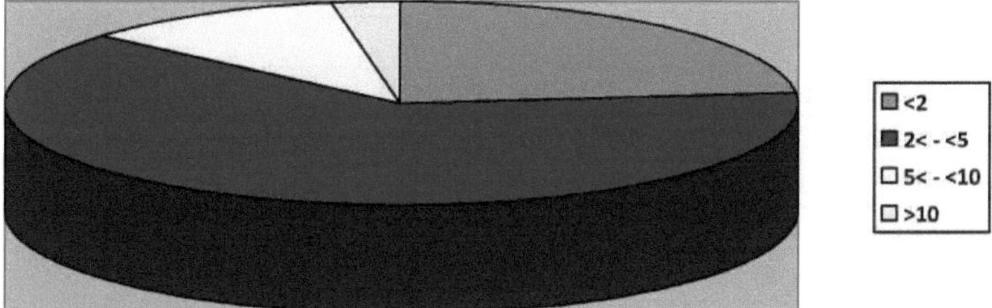

Figure 22: Distribution by size.

3) Criteria for benign tumors :

Of the 84 benign tumors the ultrasound showed:

- 76 nodular images

- 5 cystic images

- isolated ductal ectasia in 3 cases.

- **Mass:**

features		Number of cases	Percentage (%)
form	Round	43	53,1
	Oval	18	22,2
	irregular	6	7,4
	Lobulated	9	11,1
outline	Circumscribed	70	86,4
	Non–circumscribed	6	7,4
Orientation	Parallel	72	88,9
	Not parallel	9	11,1

Table 28: Distribution by characteristics of benign tumours

Echogeneity	Number of cases	Percentage (%)
Anechogen	5	5,9
Hypoechogen	60	71,4
Iso echogenic	4	4,8
Hyper echogenic	9	10,7
	6	7,14

Table 29: Echogeinicity distribution of benign tumours

The hypoechoic image was found in 60 patients, i.e. 71.4% of cases. The contours were well circumscribed in 70 cases, i.e. 86.4% of cases.

Ultrasound showed a cystic image in 5 cases, i.e. 5.9%; the image was anechoic with thin walls without vegetations in 4 cases. Only one atypical cyst was found.

Root canal ectasia in 3 cases, including one with a 5 mm endoluminal bud in one case.

- **Posterior acoustic features :**

Posterior attenuation of the echoes was noted in 10 patients, i.e. 11.9% of cases. Reinforcement was seen in 25 patients or 29.8% of cases.

- **Infiltration of the subcutaneous tissue :**

It was found in 5 cases, or 5.9% of cases.

These results allowed us to specify the ultrasound signs in favour of benignity, which are :
- Well-limited echogenic image, with long axis parallel to the skin.
- Homogeneous appearance of the internal echostructure.
- No structural change in the vicinity of the gap.
- No filling of the subcutaneous space

4) Criteria for malignancy :

Of the 146 malignant tumors the ultrasound showed:
- 145 nodular images; including 3 cases of associated simple cystic images.
- it showed a grossly inflammatory aspect in one case without any individualizable nodular image (carcinomatous mastitis).

- <u>**Mass:**</u>

features		Number of cases	percentage
Form	Round	16	11
	Oval	13	8,9
	Irregular	116	80
Contours	circumscribed	5	3,5
	Non-circumscribed	140	96,5
Orientation	Parallel	21	14,5
	Not parallel	124	85,5

Table 30: Distribution by characteristics of malignant tumours

Echogenicity	Number of cases	Percentage (%)
Hypoechogenic with irregular contours	116	80
Well-limited hypoechogenicity	28	19,4
Complex	1	0,6

Table 31: Distribution by echogeinicity

- <u>**Posterior acoustic features :**</u>
Attenuation of the beam behind the gap was noted in 65 cases, or 44.5%.

- <u>**Infiltration of the subcutaneous tissue :**</u>
It was analyzed in 73 cases, or 50%.

- <u>**Axillary adenopathy:**</u>
Ultrasound showed suspicious axillary adenopathy in 127 patients, or 87.7% of cases.

- <u>**Calcifications :**</u>
They were noted in 19 patients, i.e. 13% of cases.

From these ultrasound data, the following criteria of malignancy emerge:
- Hypoechoic, heterogeneous, irregularly contoured image with a long axis

perpendicular to the skin).
– Associated posterior attenuation

– Skin thickening in front of the lacuna.
– Presence of axillary adenopathy: increase in volume, round shape of the adenopathy, disappearance of the fatty hilum, thick asymmetric cortex and hilar hypervascularization.

5) intermediate tumors :

Intermediate tumors presented on ultrasound in both cases of complex MFK: as a cystic image with parietal thickening in one case and mild posterior enhancement of echoes in the other case.

In the case of apocrine metaplasia with simple intracanal hyperplasia lesion, the ultrasound showed a tissue image classified as ACR4 while in the case of atypical hyperplasia the ultrasound showed a homogeneous hypoechoic image well limited to the long axis parallel to the skin classified as ACR3.

In cases of intracanal papilloma, ultrasound showed ductal dilatation with an endoluminal bud classified as ACR4

The most frequent site was the upper external quadrant in 13 patients.

6) ultrasound diagnosis :

Diagnosis (n=250)	Number of cases	Percentage (%)
ACR1	2	0,8
ACR2	11	4,4
ACR3	37	14,8
ACR4	81	32,4
ACR5	119	47,6
Total	250	100

Table 32: Ultrasound diagnosis of breast tumours :

Ultrasound was normal (ACR1) in 2 cases 0.8% of cases.
It showed the existence of a benign anomaly (ACR2) in 11 cases, i.e. 4.4% of cases.
Ultrasound abnormalities were probably benign (ACR3) in 37 patients or 14.8% of cases, probably malignant in 81 patients or 32.4% and malignant in 119 patients or 47.6%.

3. HISTOLOGICAL STUDY :

A- Means :

Biopsy was performed in 172 patients, i.e. 68.8% of cases, 94.6% of which were performed in our department. Microbiopsy was performed in most cases (97%). Extemporaneous examination was performed in 38 patients while 11 cases were handled externally

In the remaining cases, the histological diagnosis was deduced from the surgical specimen in 29 patients, i.e. 11.1% of cases.

The different types of biopsies performed are illustrated below:

Means	Number of cases	percentage
Microbiopsy	153	61,2%
Surgical biopsy	19	7,6%
Extemporaneous	38	15,2%
Tumorectomy	29	11,6%
Private lumpectomy	11	4,4%

Table 33: Means of Biopsy Performed

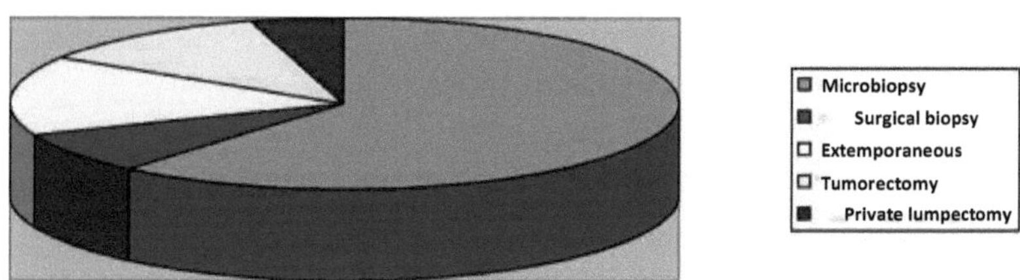

Figure 23: Means of biopsy performed

B-Histological types encountered :

Histological type	Number of cases	Percentage (%)
CCI	124	49,6
CLI	9	3,6
CCIS	8	3,2
CLIS	2	0,8
Squamous cell carcinoma	4	1,6
Metaplastic carcinoma	2	0,8
Colloidal carcinoma	1	0,4
Neuroendocrine carcinoma	2	0,8
Simple ductal hyperplasia	2	0,8
Atypical ductal hyperplasia	4	1,6
Cystic Fibrosis Mastopathy	4	1,6
Adenofibroma	70	28
Phyllodes tumor	17	6,8
Steatonecrosis nodule	1	0,4
mastitis	1	0,4
Tubular adenoma	1	0,4
total	250	100

Table 34: Definitive histological types

In our series, 124 patients had infiltrating ductal carcinoma, representing 49.6% of cases.

Lesions associated with these carcinomas have been noted:

– Outbreak of comedocarcinoma: 32 cases.

Regarding benign tumours, adenofibroma was the most frequent histological type, present in 70 patients, i.e. 28% of cases.

C–Distribution of benign and malignant and intermediate tumors:

In our series, 146 patients (58.4%) had a malignant final histological result;

Those with histologically benign tumours numbered 84, or 33.6% of cases;
While those with borderline malignancies numbered 20, or 8% of the study
sample.

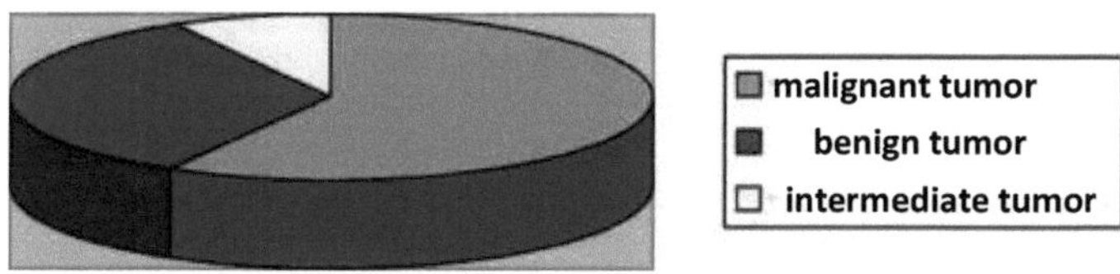

Figure 26: Distribution of breast tumours

D–Study of the histo–pronostic grade :

Histopronostic grade	Number of cases	Percentage (%)
I	17	11,6%
II	56	38,3%
III	51	35%
Not specified	22	15,1%
Total	146	100%

Table 35: Distribution by SBR histoprognostic grade for malignant tumours
The SBR grade was studied in 76 patients, or 96.20% of cases.
It showed a clear predominance of grade II and III with a percentage of 73.3%
of cases.

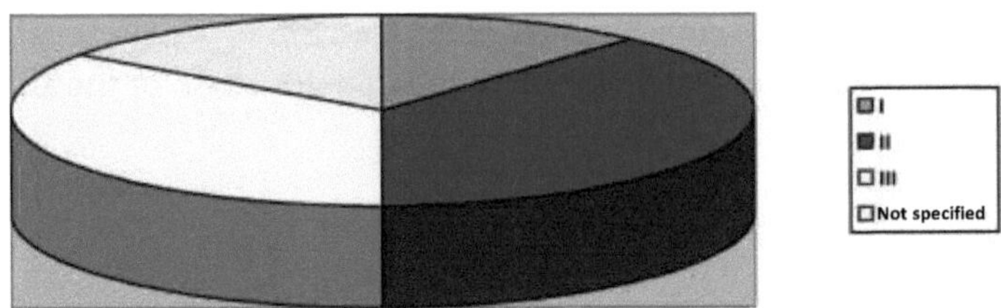

Graph 27: Distribution according to histoprognostic grade SBR for malignant tumours

E- Histological study of lymph nodes:

Histological study of lymph nodes was performed in 135 patients, i.e. 92.4% of malignant tumours.
It showed lymph node metastases in 101 patients, or 74.8% of cases.
The number of metastatic nodes ranged from 0 to 25 with an average of 6 nodes.

F-Search for hormone receptors :

Hormone receptors	Number of cases	Percentage (%)
Expression at ROE and PR	67	45,9%
Expression only at BRs	16	10,9%
Expression only in PR	6	4,1%
Lack of expression	21	14,4%
Not done	36	24,6%
TOTAL	146	100%

Table 36: Distribution of hormone receptor expression

ER = Estrogen Receptor
PR = Progesterone receptor
The immunohistochemical study showed a proliferation that expresses anti-hormone receptor antibodies in 89 cases, i.e. 61%.
It was negative in 21 patients, i.e. 14.4% of cases.

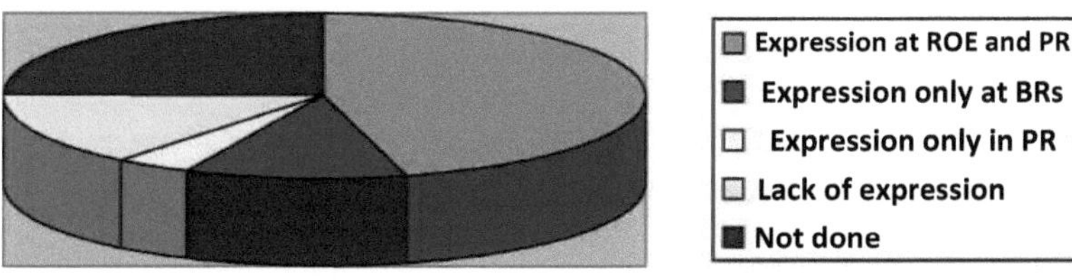

Figure 27: Distribution of hormone receptor expression

G- Vascular emboli :

The search for vascular emboli was positive in 35 patients, i.e. 24% of cases.

2.Correlations

The different correlations are listed in the tables below:

A-Clinical correlations:

Table 37: Correlation between clinical and histological findings :

clinical histology	Benin	Malin	Not conclusive
Benin	80	3	1
Malin	9	123	14
Intermediate	13	5	2

*Sensitivity: 97.03%.

Specificity: 92%.

*VPP: 93.13%.

*VPN: 94%.

B-Radio-histological correlations :
"Mammography-histology correlations:

histo-mammographic comparison:
A discrepancy between the mammographic size and the size of the lesion in pathology was found in 128 cases, i.e. 51.12%, represented mainly by infiltrating ductal carcinoma lesions.
The pathological lesion is larger than the mammographic image by 0.5 to 2.2 cm.
Among these 128 discordant cases: 79 malignant tumors (a rate of
(61.7% agreement), and 49 benign tumours (38.2% agreement).

Table 38: Correlation between mammography findings (ACR rating) and histology findings :

Mammographic lesions	Histology B	Histology M	Histology I
ACR2	12 (85,7%	0 (0%)	2 (14,3%)
ACR3	30 (79%)	5 (13,1%)	3(7,9%)
ACR4	14(23%)	44(72,1%)	3(4,9%)
ACR5	2(2,3%)	84(97,7%)	0 (0%)

Sensitivity: 93.5%.
Specificity: 86%.
 *VPP: 91.1%.
 *VPN: 93.2%.

Table 39:   Correlation between the results of mammography
(ACR classification) and histological types:

Histological type	ACR1	ACR2	ACR3	ACR4	ACR5
CCI			3	31	76
CLI			2	5	2
CCIS				3	5
CLIS			2		
Squamous cell carcinoma				3	1
Metaplastic carcinoma				2	
Colloidal carcinoma				1	
Neuroendocrine carcinoma				2	
Simple ductal hyperplasia		2			
Atypical ductal hyperplasia			4	1	
Cystic Fibrosis Mastopathy			2	2	
Adenofibroma		8	30	6	
Phyllodes tumor				7	
Steatonecrosis nodule		2			
mastitis				1	
Tubular adenoma				1	

Ultrasound – histology correlations :
***histo–echographic confrontation:**
This comparison showed a discordance in 141 cases, i.e. 56.4%.
Size was more important in histology, especially in infiltrating ductal carcinoma lesions.
The difference in measurements varied from 0.4 cm to 2 cm.

Table 40: Correlation between ultrasound findings (ACR classification) and histology findings :

Ultrasound lesions	Histology B	Histology M	Histology I
ACR2	0 (0%)	0 (0%)	13 (100%)
ACR3	32 (86,5%)	0 (0%)	5 (13,5%)
ACR4	52 (64,2%)	28 (34,6%)	1 (1,2%)
ACR5	0 (0%)	118 (99,1%)	1(0,9%)

Sensitivity: 93.89%.
Specificity: 89.7%.

*VPP: 95.4%.
  *VPN: 94.1

Table 41: Correlation between ultrasound findings (ACR classification) and histological types :

Histological type	ACR1	ACR2	ACR3	ACR4	ACR5
CCI			3	11	110
CLI			2	2	5
CCIS				3	5
CLIS			1		
Squamous cell carcinoma				3	1
Metaplastic carcinoma				2	
Colloidal carcinoma				1	
Neuroendocrine carcinoma				2	
Simple ductal hyperplasia		2			
Atypical ductal hyperplasia		4		1	
Cystic Fibrosis Mastopathy			2	2	
Adenofibroma			22	48	
Phyllodes tumor			4	11	2
Steatonecrosis nodule			2		
mastitis				1	
Tubular adenoma				1	

III. Discussion

1- Epidemiology:

Breast cancer is the most common tumor in women in Morocco and the second in the world by its incidence, it represents the first cause of female mortality by cancer. Statistically, it is estimated that one out of ten women living to 80 years old will develop breast cancer during her lifetime.

In Morocco, between 30,000 and 45,000 people are affected by cancer each year according to official information from the 2001 statistics of the Sidi Mohammed Ben Abdellah National Institute of Oncology in Rabat, which represents 101.7 new cases per year per 100,000 inhabitants.

Breast cancer is the first female cancer with an incidence of between 12,000 and 15,000 new cases detected each year, of which 53% of cases are in urban areas and 73% in rural areas where the disease is discovered at an advanced stage. (1)

This incidence has increased in Morocco, as in the whole world, by more than 60% from 1975 to 1995. In fact, the number of cases doubled between 1985 (417 cases) and 2002 (987 cases) (2), while the increase in mortality was more moderate (+8%). This is also the case in France, where the rate doubled between 1980 and 2005, with mortality remaining stable and then beginning to decrease since the end of the 1990s (-1.3% over the period 2000-2005).

These increases are partly explained by several factors, including the ageing of the population and the widespread use of screening, which allows more cancers to be diagnosed at an earlier stage (2).

78% of breast cancers occur after the age of 50 and only 6% in women under 40. However, there is currently a tendency for this cancer to become younger.

Worldwide, breast cancer is responsible for more than one million new cases per year and nearly 410,000 female deaths in 2002 (3). Consequently, it represents a real public health problem

In our series during these two years 2011-2012, breast pathology comes first in gynecology hospitalizations with a frequency of 39.6%.

II - Clinical study :

A- Circumstances of discovery

1- Tumor:

On self-examination, it is the main revealing sign (4, 5, 6). It is seen in 65% to 80% of patients (5).

In our study, the nodule was the revealing sign in 96.8% of cases.

2- Pain:

According to the literature, 4.8% of breast tumors have been found to have mastodynia (7)

In our series, this rate is 0.4% of patients with breast pain.

3- Nipple discharge:

Nipple discharge represents 3 to 5% of pathologies breast. (5)

In our series, nipple discharge was observed in 2 patients; in only one case was it the sign of call leading the patient to consult and in the other cases this sign was presented in association with other signs.

4- Skin and nipple changes:

According to the literature, it is observed in 5 to 7% of cases (8,9). In our series, skin changes were noted in 14% of cases.

5- Isolated axillary adenopathy It has been found that patients rarely consult for one or more isolated axillary adenopathies (5,6).

In our series, none of our patients consulted for isolated axillary adenopathy but associated with other signs (most often a breast nodule) in 37.6% of cases.

B- Clinical examination :

1-Breast Examination:

Inspection :

Malignant inflammatory lesions account for 1-5% of cancerous lesions, while benign inflammatory lesions are rare, presenting 1% (10).

In our series, inflammatory manifestations were present in 9.6% of tumors.

Palpation:

The superior-external quadrant was the most frequent location in our series, which is consistent with the results of other series (11,12).

2- Examination of lymph nodes : (30,25, 26).

In our series, 37.6% of cases had clinically palpable adenopathy.

3-Examination of the contralateral breast :

Synchronous bilateral involvement is rare, whether benign or malignant, but examination of the other breast should not be neglected, as 10% of bilateral cancers occur immediately (5, 6, 11, 13).

The examination of our patients showed bilateral palpable involvement in 4.3% of cases. We did not consider subclinical lesions of the contralateral breast. **4-General examination:**

It allows us to look for defects and metastases that may contraindicate the necessary treatments.

According to the literature, 5 to 10% of breast cancers are metastatic from the start (5, 7, 11).

In our series, 6.4% of patients hospitalized had metastatic cancer at the time of diagnosis. The reason for hospitalization was either histological confirmation.

III-Radiological study :

A-Mammography :

Mammography remains the fundamental examination in breast imaging. It requires a perfect technique to analyze the radiological signals. The positive predictive value of suspicious radiological images varies according to the type and shape of the abnormality analysed (14, 15, 16). (14, 15, 16)

Mammographic images are classified according to the degree of suspicion of their pathological nature. The BIRADS (Breast Imaging Reporting and Data System) classification of the ACR (American College of Radiology) recommended by the ANAES (Agence Nationale d'Accréditation et d'Evaluation en santé) is currently used.

<u>**1-Benign tumors :**</u>

In our series, they were manifested by a rounded or oval opacity, with regular contours in 89.4% of cases.

- **Adenofibroma :**

Most commonly, it is a round, homogeneously dense, evenly contoured, well circumscribed opacity with or without lobulations (11, 17, 18).

In our series, 30 of the 70 adenofibromas had the characteristics described above and were all classified as ACR3. 8 cases were classified as ACR2 and 6 cases were classified as ACR4 mainly because of their heterogeneous content.

In 40 cases, mammography was performed in young girls with dense breasts, and the diagnosis of adenofibroma was made by ultrasound.

Old, hyalinized fibroadenomas may become irregular, with ill-defined contours, sometimes with the appearance of micro calcifications. These micro calcifications observed are of various shapes, thick, popcorn-shaped or linear, punctiform, granular or pleomorphic, and the lesion may also be completely or partially calcified in a semicircle or oyster shell (17, 19, 20).

- **<u>Phyllodes tumor:</u>**

Produces a large (3-40 cm) oval or polycyclic opacity with regular contours and no axillary extension or microcalcifications (19,21).

For VERHAGHE, two radiological characteristics should make one think of a phyllodes tumour: the polycyclic appearance and the clear contour in some places, blurred in others (18, 22, 23).

In our series and among the 17 phyllodes tumors present, 7 were classified as ACR 4 and in no case was the opacity accompanied by micro calcifications, which is consistent with the literature. For the other cases of phyllodes tumors, mammography was not performed due to either the young age of the patient in 9 cases or the inflammatory nature in 1 case.

- **Ductal ectasia**

It has been shown to be linear calcifications oriented towards the nipple, intracanal, not to be confused with type V calcifications indicative of cancer (19,24).

• **Fibrocystic Dystrophy or Mastopathy**

Cysts larger than 3 mm in diameter appear as round or oval, homogeneous opacities with clear boundaries, all the more individualizable as the breasts are fatty (ACR2). They are sometimes masked by adjacent dystrophic structures (ACR2), indicating a suspicious appearance (ACR4) (11, 19), hence the need for comparative analysis of mammographic images (24, 25).

In our series and among the 4 cases of fibrocystic mastopathy 2 cases were classified ACR 4.

Mastitis :

Mammographic translation showed an ACR4 appearance.

According to the literature, it is an entity of non-specific radiological translation and can be benign or radiologically malignant. (26,27,28)

Intracanal papilloma:

In the form of a discreetly echogenic nodule within a dilated duct or tubular duct, surrounded by an echogenic mantle (19,26). Distal papillomas in particular, on the other hand, are mammographically occult in over 50% of cases (29). On the other hand, some papillomas may progress to fibrosis and calcify. The microcalcifications observed may then be punctiform, polymorphic or flaky, or even suspicious looking.

Other

Cytosteatonecrosis : (26,30) In recent forms where fibrous reorganization has not yet occurred, mammography shows a radiolucent mass with a thicker or thinner contour, the outer side of which is sometimes spiculated.

In our study, the cytosteonecrosis nodules were classified as ACR2

- **Hamartoma**: manifests as a voluminous homogeneous opacity that is non-specific in 30% of cases, or heterogeneous (most often typical) depending on its content (19).

2- Malignant tumors :

Mammography is more effective after the menopause. Typically, breast cancer appears as a dense, stellate, irregularly contoured opacity in which microcalcifications can sometimes be found, and very often there is skin thickening opposite the lesion (03, 21, 26, 31, 32).

In our series, mammography showed an opacity with irregular contours in 54.2% of the cases of malignant tumors, of which the stellate form represented 39.9% of the cases with which micro calcifications were associated in 38% of the cases and the majority of which were classified as ACR5 (60%), and skin thickening was associated in 19.6% of the cases

Using the ACR BI RADS language: 82.2% of breast cancer cases were classified as ACR5 or ACR4 with a predominance of ACR5 (54.2%).

- Carcinoma in situ

<u>a- Ductal carcinoma in situ (DCIS):</u>

Isolated foci of microcalcifications (presence of at least five microcalcifications in 1cm3) are the source of the diagnosis of the majority of CCIS in over 65% of cases (33).

Two types of microcalcifications can be described (33, 34, 35,36):

- Rather round and irregular fine or coarse granular type, frequently found in non-comedogenic CCIS.

- Vermicular, branched and polymorphic type, more representative of comedocarcinomas in situ.

The clustering of these calcifications, the triangular shape of the focus or its angular contours and its mamelon-like orientation, reflect their intracanal location (33, 37,38).

CCIS may be revealed by other mammographic features: nodular opacity, architectural distortion, and increased density (10).

In our series, 8 cases of CCIS were present, 5 of which appeared on mammography as irregularly contoured opacities graded ACR5 without a focus of microcalcifications. In the remaining three cases, mammography showed isolated microcalcifications all classified as ACR4.

<u>b- Lobular carcinoma in situ (LCIS):</u>

According to DIANNE GEORGIAN-SMITH, CLIS is characterized by clustered, high-density, punctiform or polymorphic calcifications that tend to be round and almost always less than or equal to 0.5 mm in size (39, 40).

In our series,   2 cases of CLIS presented as foci of microcalcifications classified as ACR3.

- Invasive carcinoma :

<u>a- Invasive ductal carcinoma (IDC):</u>

It represents 75% of round cancers. It most often corresponds to a well-limited opacity with irregular contours(32).

For a diagnosis of suspicion, it is necessary to be very attentive to a loss of regularity of contour, to the existence of numerous micro calcifications, of galactophoric disposition and of high type according to the Curie classification (41). Stellate appearance was noted in 52% (10).

In our series this aspect was found in a proportion of 52.05%.

In our series, the ICC was a round or oval opacity with irregular contours, or stellate in 63.01% of cases, with associated atypical micro calcifications in 26% of cases.

In 61.3% of the cases the mammogram showed a lesion classified as ACR5, and in 33.06% of the cases of CCI the mammogram was classified as ACR4.

Only 3 cases were classified as ACR 3, i.e. 2.4% of all CCI cases. These were breast tumours handled privately or in a health facility and for which the ultrasound mammography was performed on an outpatient basis.

<u>b- Invasive lobular carcinoma (ILC):</u>

It is often difficult to diagnose on mammography, and nearly half of the cases are manifested by a nodular opacity with regular contours without suspicious microcalcifications simulating a fibroadenoma (4, 35).

Other authors say that CLI often results in stellate opacity, sometimes in architectural distortion or only in calcifications

(37), as in our series, where two CLIs appeared as round spiculated opacities graded ACR5 but without a focus of microcalcifications. Five cases presented as a lesion graded ACR4 and two cases as ACR3.

There are no mammographic features to distinguish CLI from CCI.

<u>**c- metaplastic carcinoma :**</u>

Mammographic features are not specific. The mammographic signs reported as suggestive are the hyperdensity of the mass and the absence of microcalcifications (24). The same appearance was found in cases of metaplastic carcinoma in our series, which was found as a bilobed opacity with regular contours.

Some studies show the possible association of squamous metaplasia with adenocarcinomas, the frequency of this association is estimated by FISCHER at 3.6% (75) and at 0.5% by TOIKKANEN (41).

The rare cases where proliferation is pure have been reported by ARFFMAN (41) BOGOMOLETZ (42), SHOUSHA (43) and JIN (44), <u>**d- Mucinous carcinoma:**</u> It is a well-defined circumscribed opacity with lobulated, sometimes discretely spiculated, contours. Microcalcifications are very rare and not typical (12, 20, 21).

In our series, colloid carcinoma found in a 50-year-old patient manifested on mammography as a lesion classified as ACR 4.

<u>**e- Medullary carcinoma :**</u>

It can be multifocal. It corresponds to a round or oval opacity with sometimes blurred contours, with a comet tail appearance. It is never a stellar image (12). No case was seen in our study **f- Other :**

- Papillary carcinoma: corresponds to a well-circumscribed round opacity, almost always endocanal (12).

- Tubular carcinoma: rarely round (10% of cases), but most often stellate. Microcalcifications and architectural distortion may be seen (32).

• **Breast sarcoma :**

The mammographic appearance is often characteristic. It corresponds to a dense, rounded or oval or polycyclic opacity with a regular contour, sometimes associated with intra-tumoral calcifications that are often coarse.

Importantly, it has no stellar extension (25, 26).

In our study, the only sarcoma encountered was a phyllodes sarcoma, which translated mammographically into a large opacity measuring 12 cm in long axis, with a homogeneous poly-lobed watery tone classified as ACR4, without any suspicious micro-calcifications.

- **Breast lymphoma :**

It is most often a breast location of a known non-Hodgkin's lymphoma. It presents as a more or less limited round opacity, which is never stellate and without microcalcifications. This deceptively reassuring appearance is present in most cases (17, 18).

- **Breast metastases**

The mammographic appearance is that of well-circumscribed opacities that are often multifocal (12).

3-Atypical hyperplasia:

There are no pathognomonic radiological features of simple or atypical ductal hyperplasia. In most cases, the hyperplastic foci are not large enough to cause a mammographic abnormality.

Rubin et al. (45), foci of microcalcifications constitute up to 80% of the mammographic appearance of atypical hyperplasia and over 60% of that of simple epithelial hyperplasia.

In Legal's series, which is often used as a reference, atypical hyperplasia is associated with foci of microcalcifications of type 2, 3 or 4 according to Le Gal, but never type 1 or 5; in our series, 4 cases of atypical hyperplasia resulted in microcalcifications classified as ACR3 of the BI RADS type 2 classification according to Legal.

Other mammographic abnormalities that may be associated with atypical hyperplasia are architectural distortions (23%), masses (9%), and no abnormality is found in 9% of cases. (29)

8- Ultrasound :

It is becoming part of the diagnostic tripod to the extent that it is an extension of palpation and an indispensable complement to mammography (11, 25). This examination is particularly indicated when the breasts are radiologically dense, and is the technique of choice for young women (21).

1- Benign tumors :

In our series, ultrasound showed a hypoechoic image with regular contours in 86.4%

of cases, and with a long axis parallel to the skin in 85.7% of cases, and a cystic image in 3.2% of cases.

• Adenofibroma :

Ultrasound most often shows the fibroadenoma as a round or oval image, with regular contours and a long axis parallel to the skin, often homogeneous hypoechoic, providing an excellent medium for sound wave propagation, without attenuation (34).

The fibroadenoma is not deformable under the probe, very well seen in the fibrous tissue.

In our study, the fibroadenoma appeared as a well-limited homogeneous hypoechoic image in 31.4% of cases.

It should be noted that fibroadenoma, which is sensitive to hormonal impregnation, presents different characteristics according to age. (34)

• Phyllodes tumor:

The image is oval or poly-lobed, homogeneous hypoechoic, sometimes calcified with heterogeneous echostructure, with more or less clear boundaries.

However, a fine ultrasound scan will show small cystic lesions at the edge of or inside a solid nodule (34).

In our study out of the 17 cases of phyllodes tumors 4 were homogeneous hypoechoic oval with two of them calcified classified as ACR3. And 11 cases were sonographically translated as a lobulated image classified as ACR4.

• Intracanal papilloma:

As a discrete echogenic nodule within a dilated duct or tubular duct, surrounded by an echogenic sleeve (35,39).

It should be noted that ultrasound cannot distinguish between intracystic carcinomas and papillomas.

• Fibrocystic mastopathy:

It appears as an anechoic, round or oval image with high contrast. The borders are sharp, fine and regular, but there are sometimes intra-cystic septa.

When fibrosis predominates, it may be accompanied by fine posterior attenuation bundles which, when in close proximity, may mimic a suspicious image (11, 34)

In our series, it was manifested by a well circumscribed, thin-walled, slightly heterogeneous anechoic image classified as ACR3 in 50% of cases and with irregular borders classified as ACR4 in 2 cases.

- **Other :**
- **Intramammary ganglion**: as an oval hypoechoic lacuna with a hyperechoic centre (19).
- **Lipoma**: Ultrasound is unnecessary because the contrast of the lipoma with normal fat lobules may be very low (19).
- **Hamartoma**: ultrasound shows alternating hyperechoic and hypoechoic areas in the shape of a sausage slice (19).

2- Malignant tumors :

Malignant lesions seen on ultrasound are essentially invasive, even when small, because of its poor perception of microcalcifications (34).

In our series, ultrasound showed a hypoechoic image of irregular shape in 79.4% of cases, associated with a heterogeneous image in 19.9% of cases, with the major axis perpendicular to the skin plane in 85% of cases.

- **Carcinoma In situ**

Ultrasound is hardly involved in the diagnosis of carcinoma in situ (35).

In our series, all 8 CCIS appeared as images classified as ACR4 or ACR5.

- **Invasive carcinoma**

- Invasive ductal carcinoma

It often appears as a poorly limited image, with a heterogeneous appearance of the internal echostructure, more or less hypoechoic, with its long axis perpendicular to the skin or with an axis of more than 20° with the skin (19).

The shadow cone is present in 41% of cases of infiltrating ductal carcinoma, but there may be posterior enhancement which should not lead to a diagnosis of benignity (17).

In our series, ITC was a heterogeneous hypoechoic image, with irregular contours in 84.9% of cases, with a shadow cone in 51% of cases.

In ACR termology, of the 124 cases of ICC, 110 (88.7%) were classified as

ACR5, 11 (8.9%) were classified as ACR4 and only 3 cases were classified as ACR3. This means that 97.5% of the invasive ductal carcinomas in our study were classified as ACR4 or ACR5, which is consistent with the BIRADS ACR classification data which gives these two categories a significant positive predictive value of malignancy exceeding 95% for lesions classified as ACR5

- __Invasive lobular carcinoma :__

Infiltrating lobular carcinoma is characterized on ultrasound by a hypoechoic, irregularly shaped lesion with uncircumscribed contours that may be indistinct, micro lobulated or speculated. These boundaries appear as an echogenic halo that corresponds to a transition zone without any sharp delineation. This lesion may be wider than it is tall and posterior attenuation is often present, especially when the lesion is very fibrous or stellate on mammography. In our series, two cases of CLI fit this description and were classified as ACR4, while 5 cases were classified as ACR5. For Skaane (100), one sign is particularly important: the hyper-echogenic crown present in 81% of cases.

There are atypical forms that manifest as a poorly defined hyperechoic image that does not meet the criteria for malignancy (18).

c- __metaplastic carcinoma :__

Breast ultrasound can show solid and cystic areas, which correspond to foci of necrosis, haemorrhage and cystic degeneration, hence the need to evoke the diagnosis of metaplastic carcinoma in the presence of a breast nodule with a cystic component (10, 11) In our series, ultrasound, in both cases, showed a heterogeneous mass classified as ACR 4.

- __Mucinous carcinoma :__

The sonographic appearance is that of a hypoechoic image with an irregular margin and a shadow cone, sometimes isoechoic.

In fact, echogenicity depends on the type of mucinous carcinoma (8, 13).

- __Medullary carcinoma__ :

It has a benign appearance on ultrasound, with a depth to width ratio of less than one (32).

- Tubular carcinoma

As a hypoechoic image without specificity (32).

• Breast sarcoma :

It can give the appearance of a homogeneous image with regular contours evoking a benign lesion.

The search for central necrosis suggests malignancy (16).

The only sarcoma in our study is a phyllodes sarcoma which, according to the literature, is seen on ultrasound as a single or multiple heterogeneous hypoechoic mass with generally well-defined contours. These tumours cannot be differentiated on ultrasound from fibroadenomas or from well circumscribed malignant tumours. However, phyllodes sarcoma should be considered when a well-vascularized and well-circumscribed solid-cystic tumor is found (14). This was the case with our phyllodes carcinoma classified as ACR4.

• Malignant lymphoma :

It often appears on ultrasound as a well-limited homogeneous or heterogeneous hyperechoic nodular image (26,15).

V- HISTOLOGICAL STUDY :

A- Means :

1- Extemporaneous :

It is one of the pillars of the diagnostic workup and its interest is to guide the extent of the surgical procedure.

The concordance of the preoperative diagnosis with that made on paraffin sections is 90% overall for infiltrating malignant tumours (24).

On the other hand, there is almost unanimous agreement not to perform an extemporaneous examination on an isolated focus of microcalcifications, without a palpable lesion. In practice, the study of these specimens always requires the inclusion of numerous samples (29).

In our series, the extemporaneous examination was performed in 15.2% of the cases, of which 4.6% were in favour of in situ or inconclusive, whereas the definitive histological examination was in favour of malignancy, hence the resumption of these patients in 100% of cases.

2- <u>Biopsy :</u>

It allows the diagnosis, histopronostic grade and hormone receptors of the tumor (13). The degree of reliability of the diagnosis of malignancy is around 90% (24).

In our series, the biopsy was performed in 68.8% of cases with a degree of reliability of 93.4%.

B- Macroscopic study :

Macroscopic examination is essential in determining which specimen to examine (29). It consists of assessing the tumour size in all three dimensions, consistency, colour and precise topography, in particular in relation to the nearest resection limits. These requirements include marking of the resection limits and radiography of the parts when they contain microcalcifications (31).

C- Histological types of benign tumors :

1- <u>Adenofibroma or fibroadenoma: (19, 32, 33, 34)</u>

It is a fibroepithelial proliferation occurring preferentially in young women, with a frequency of 15.7%. It is bilateral in 10-15% of cases, and there is usually no recurrence. The risk of further degeneration or association with cancer is rare (0.1%). According to Dupont and Page the relative risk of degeneration of complex fibroadenomas is 3.1, and it increases to 3.72 in case of a family history of breast cancer.

In our series, it represents 28% of the cases; second in order of frequency of all the tumors and first among the benign tumors

2- <u>Phyllodes tumor: (38, 39, 41) :</u>

It represents 0.3 to 4% of breast tumours, with 4 stages from benign to malignant (sarcoma) according to the CONTESSO classification.

Thus, the absence of a peripheral capsule explains the high risk of local recurrence.

In our series, there were 17 cases of phyllodes tumor or 6.8% of cases. Microbiopsy was in favor of adenofibroma.

3- Adenoma: (30, 36)

This is a rare benign tumour, made up of pure epithelial proliferation, forming a milky adenoma in young women or tubular adenoma. This lesion should not be confused with a carcinoma, especially during the extemporaneous examination, but it should be noted that a carcinoma can be observed on an adenoma.

In our series, its frequency is about 0.4%.

4- Papilloma: (29, 39)

It is a proliferating lesion developed from the galactophore duct, of papillary architecture, it is either unique (solitary or central papilloma) presenting 70 to 90% of cases, or multiple (papillomatosis) with a frequency of 10 to 30%, or translating an erosive adenomatosis.

In our series, one case of intracavitary papilloma was found.

5- Simple cystic fibrosis: (30, 33, 39) :

A very vague term that encompasses a number of benign, non-cancerous, non-inflammatory histological lesions. It is the most common condition in the breast (66.3%). These dystrophies combine cysts by ductal dilatation and epithelial hyperplasia in the galactophoric tree, the latter comprising 3 aspects: epitheliosis or papillomatosis, adenosis and the proliferative centre of aschoff.

In our study, it represents 1.6% of cases.

6- Hamartome: (27, 33)

It is in fact a well-limited pseudotumor lesion, consisting of the proliferation of three tissues: connective, epithelial and fatty. It represents 1.7% of tumors.

No cases were found in our series.

7- Lipoma: (14)

It corresponds to a benign proliferation of fatty tissue.

In our series, no lipoma was observed

8- Other : (30, 39, 44)

- Ductal ectasia or plasma cell mastitis: characterized by galactophoric dilatation associated with pericanal fibrosis. The incidence of this condition is 1 in 10 to 15 breast dysplasias. It represents 5.66% of cases in our series. - Intramammary ganglion: it represents 1% of benign tumours, there is no case in our series.

- Granulomatous mastitis: there are less than 100 cases published in the literature and in our series, no case was found.

- Conjunctival tumours: these are very rare, and four particular entities must be distinguished: haemangioma, myoblastoma, fibromatosis and leiomyoma.

D- Histological types of malignant tumors :

1- <u>Carcinoma:</u>

It accounts for 90% of malignant breast tumours.

- Carcinoma in situ :

    J Ductal carcinoma in situ: (13, 14, 41, 42, 43)

It represents a histological variant which is comedocarcinoma.

The majority of ductal carcinomas in situ become infiltrative. They can colonize the milk shaft up to the nipple (Paget's disease).

In our series, it represents 3.2% of cases.

    J Lobular carcinoma in situ: (24, 44, 45)

It does not develop directly into invasive cancer but it is an indicator of high risk, multiple or bilateral locations are common. It represents 0.7% of cancers. It was found in 0.8% of cases in our study.

- <u>Invasive carcinoma :</u>

    J Invasive ductal carcinoma : (23,41)

It is the most frequent form of breast carcinoma, about 80%. In our series, it represented 49.6%.

Some invasive ductal carcinomas are associated with a predominantly intracanal component, this form represents about 5% of all invasive carcinomas. In our series, it represented 9.8% of cases.

    J Invasive lobular carcinoma : (27,31)

It represents 4% of invasive carcinomas. In our series, it represents 1.25% of cases. Invasive lobular carcinomas are associated with lobular carcinomas in situ in 70% of cases, they are often diffuse and multifocal, hence the indication for breast MRI.

J Medullary carcinoma : (31)

No cases of medullary carcinoma were diagnosed in our study.

J Metaplastic carcinoma : (15,16)

Metaplastic carcinomas of the breast are rare tumours, representing less than 1% of invasive carcinomas of the breast (43). 2 cases, i.e. 0.8% of all the tumours in our study, were identified.

J Papillary carcinoma : (24, 31)

It represents only 0.3% of invasive carcinomas.

J Mucinous carcinoma (8,13):

It represents only 1% of all invasive breast cancers, in our study it represents 0.6% of breast carcinomas.

J Other invasive carcinomas : (13,15)

They are rare, adenoid or cylindroid, carcinoid, apocrine, cribriform, metaplastic.

• <u>Paget's disease : (13)</u>

It represents 2% of cancers, only 2 cases were noted in our series. It corresponds to the extension to the nipple of an underlying ductal or lobular breast carcinoma.

2- <u>Primary non-epithelial malignant lesions : (9)</u>

They are rare and account for about 1% of all breast cancers.

Four histological types are distinguished:

- Phyllodes sarcoma and which presented 0.8% of cases in our series.

- Mesenchymal sarcoma.

- Angiosarcoma.

- Malignant non-Hodgkin's lymphoma of the breast.

E- Histopronostic grade :

Different kinds of histopronostic grading have been proposed for a long time, the most used is the modified Scarff Bloom and Richardson (SBR) histopronostic grading.

This grading takes into account three characteristics: degree of differentiation, anisonucleosis and mitotic activity. It allows tumours to be classified into three grades, I, II, III, with increasingly unfavourable prognoses. This grading can be applied to all infiltrating carcinomas of the breast with the exception of the typical medullary forms (31).

Table 33: Proportion of different grades in the literature

authors SBR	I (%)	II (%)	III(%)
Touboul (81)	12,07	62,07	25,86
Calitchi (12)	20,47	46,45	33,08
Broet (8)	25,27	59,08	15,65
Otmezguine (67)	17,07	56,09	26,84
Our series	11,6	38,3	35,5

In our series, there is a predominance of grade II, and this is consistent with the literature as shown in the table.

F- Histological status of lymph nodes:

Locoregional lymph node involvement is the most representative metastatic mode of a carcinoma's aggressiveness and the main feature considered to predict outcome.

This characteristic is not continuous and various increasingly unfavourable subgroups can be distinguished according to whether there are no N- metastatic nodes, 1 to 3 N+, 4 to 10 N+, or more than 10 N+ (27, 33).

In our series, the number of metastatic nodes ranged from 0 to 25 with an average of 6.

Node invasion was assessed in 74.8% of cases, and according to the literature, it is estimated at 25-40%.

In the presence of palpable axillary nodes, the probability of histological lymph node involvement is 65-80% (24).

G- Hormone receptors :

The value of the hormone receptor assay was analyzed by studying

PETO, which has clarified their prognostic and therapeutic values in breast cancer (15).

The biochemical assay is a reference method that has entered routine practice, based on a cytosolic assay of hormone receptors, whereas the immunohistochemical method is based on an antigen-antibody reaction supported by histological sections (31).

In the literature, the concordance between the two techniques gives fairly similar results.

However, it should be emphasized that immunohistochemistry is able to ensure that the section slice does indeed contain an invasive carcinoma, thus avoiding false positives obtained by biochemical assay due to the presence of receptors in normal tissues and intracanal carcinomatous structures (31).

In our series, hormone receptor testing was positive in 60.9% of cases and negative in 14.4%.

VI- Clinical-histological comparison

The clinical examination of the breast is too often neglected in favour of complementary examinations.

Although the clinical examination can never formally confirm the diagnosis, which is left to the histological examination, in most cases it allows a strong suspicion to be raised. In addition, the clinical examination helps to guide the assessment of extension.

An anatomical-clinical comparison is necessary to highlight the diagnostic value of the clinical examination.

Table 49   Representation of the results of the clinical confrontation-Histological.

clinical histology	Benin	Malin	Not conclusive	Total
Benin	80 (78,4%)	3(2,3%)	1(5,9%)	84
Malin	9(8,8%)	123(93,9%)	14(82,3%)	146
Intermediate	13(12,7%)	5(3,8%)	2(11,8%)	20
Total	102	131	17	250

According to the analysis of this clinical-histological comparison, we note that among the lesions supposed to be benign on clinical examination 78.4% (80 cases) are actually benign on histology, while 8.8% are malignant.

In the second clinical group (131 cases) where the lesions are considered malignant 93.9% (123 cases) are actually malignant on histology, while 2.3% (3 cases) are benign and 3.8% are borderline malignant.

In the third group where the clinic was inconclusive (1 case), 5.9% were benign and 82.3% (14 cases) were malignant.

If we consider each group of tumors separately, the results can be presented as follows:

Of the 84 benign tumours, we note :

- In 80 cases the diagnosis is concordant;
- In 1 case the diagnosis is not concordant;
- And in 3 cases the diagnosis is misleading.

- Of the 146 malignant tumours, we note :
- In 123 cases the diagnosis is concordant;
- In 14 cases the diagnosis is not concordant;
- And in 9 cases the diagnosis is misleading.

In the case of malignant tumors, the clinical-histological diagnostic concordance is more important than for benign tumors.

The clinic makes more misleading cases in malignant tumors than in malignant tumors.

For all the benign and malignant tumours out of the 250 tumours, the clinic was concordant in 203 cases, i.e. a concordance rate of 81.2%.

If we take all the cases studied, the concordance index is 0.69. This represents a strong agreement between the two parameters, testifying to the important diagnostic value of the clinic in the field of breast pathology.

In the literature:

Table 52: Representation of the results of the anatomical-clinical comparisons in the literature

Clinical diagnosis (Author)	Concordance rate
Lansac (156)	75%
Helene zadeh (157)	79,10%
Gynecology Clinic of Lyon (157)	82%
Pivard and Roussignol (158)	75,14%
F.Moussaoui (157)	80,2%
Schaaps and Colin (158)	52%
A. Bremond	66%
Our series	81,2%

Comparing the rate of clinical-histological concordance found in our series with the results of other series represented in the table above, we note that the concordance is very important in our series, and remains close to that of the gynecological clinic in Lyon (82%).

As for the series where the clinical examination was inconclusive, the series by Schaaps and Colin has the lowest concordance index (52%). All the authors strive to increase the performance of the clinical examination. This also fits our environment, especially since in our series, and despite the high concordance index, the clinic has recorded misleading cases in malignant pathology, which even if they are not very frequent, must push us to improve our performance even more as clinicians.

VII-HISTO-RADIOLOGICAL COMPARISON OF BREAST TUMOURS :

A- Size :

1- Histo-mammographic comparison :

The comparison between the mammographic signal and the pathological data is carried out on the size of the lesion whether it is located on the main part or on a recut.

Lesion measurements are considered to be concordant if they differ by less than 2 mm on both axes (39).

A discrepancy between the size of the mammographic signal and that of the pathological lesion was found in 32.2%, represented in more than half of the cases (55%) by lesions of ductal carcinoma in situ; 20% of infiltrating lobular carcinomas; 15% of infiltrating ductal carcinomas and 5% of lobular carcinoma in situ. The pathological lesion is more important than the mammographic appearance (39).

This notion has already been reported by HOLLAND. Focal or diffuse pathological lesions of atypical hyperplasia, ductal carcinoma in situ and lobular carcinoma in situ were found in 35% of cases (19, 28).

There is a direct relationship between size and invasive microscopic features, such as high nuclear grade, necrosis, microinvasion and multifocality.

A difference in size of more than 2 cm between the mammographic estimate and the anatomical lesion is found in 8% of ductal comedocarcinomas in situ, and in 47% of cribriform ductal carcinomas in situ (28).

In our series, the discrepancy between the size of the mammographic signal and that of the pathological lesion is present in 51.2% of cases, particularly in infiltrating ductal carcinoma with a higher proportion of measurements ranging from 0.5 cm to 2.2 cm for malignant tumors.

This allows us to state that a pathological study focused on the radiological signal does not allow us to evaluate the extent of the malignant pathology.

The mammo-histological correlation is concordant for benign pathology in several studies (36, 39, 40). A variability of proportions is observed. In our series, the proportion reached 61.8% for all benign tumours.

2- **Histo-echographic confrontation:**

Ultrasound measurements of the tumor image including the "halo" better reflect the true size of the tumor in pathology (19, 40).

SKAANE (37) reports a close agreement between tumour size and pathology and that of ultrasound with a correlation coefficient of 0.69 (95% confidence limit 0.54 to 0.79). Thus the predictive value of ultrasound measurements is not significant for infiltrating lobular carcinoma.

The pathological diagnosis of lesions less than or equal to 10 mm in size is benign in 48.4%, malignant in 43.8% and atypical hyperplasia in 7.8% of cases (39).

These data are not correlated with our series where we found a discordance between the size in pathology and that of the ultrasound at a proportion of 56.40% on all the tumors.

8- **Benign tumors :**

1- Correlation between mammography and histology :

The benign pathological diagnosis correlated with the mammographic appearance is shown in the following table.

Table 53: Distribution by mammographic appearance

Authors	Nodule	Calcifications	Architectural disorganization	Other signs
CHOPIER (15)	12	42	0	0
GOLLENTZ (37)	21	42	6	0
Our series	57	4	4	3

According to these studies, the nodular appearance is the second most frequent mammographic appearance (25.38%), corresponding in the majority of cases to a regular opacity with clear contours, rounded, oval or poly-lobed (29). In our series this aspect was the first in order of frequency (67.8%), and in accordance with the data in the literature the well circumscribed opacity was found in 58.3% of cases of benign tumours.

Microcalcifications correlate with bilateral complex benign pathology involving fibrocystic mastopathy lesions , fibrotic fibroadenomas, sclerosing adenosis and papillomatous formations (29). The importance of calcifications in mammography stems from their character as a prominent sign, taking into account the size, number, shape, grouping and distribution of calcifications (30).

The semiological aspects of calcifications suggestive of benignity are well defined (36) :

- Round, annular, multiple calcifications, cysts and microcysts in particular.
- Cup-shaped calcifications.
- Coarse intracanal calcifications of the ectasia.
- Very extensive, even bilateral, fine calcifications, "mastoses".

Other authors (24) report that the type I microcalcifications described by LE GAL (ACR2) are always benign.

Thus, the histo-mammographic correlation is total for benign pathology since in all cases, the mammographic aspect corresponds to a lesion characterized in pathology.

The mammographic appearance considered to be strictly correlated with atypical hyperplasia is that of microcalcifications. HELVIE and STOMPER report respective figures of 34 and 35% of atypical hyperplasia discovered incidentally at a distance from the radiological signal (19).

According to the literature, mammography is capable of evoking benign mastopathy, with a sensitivity of 88% and a specificity of 76% (12).

2- Correlation between ultrasound and histology:

Assigning a breast tumor to be benign is usually easy by studying its echostructure.

Ultrasound is used to carefully analyse hypoechoic tissue images. It helps to identify fibroadenomas with their regular contours and their long axis parallel to the cutaneous-muscular plane (14).

LE TREUT (19) reports that a well circumscribed, round or oval appearance, a homogeneous echostructure and posterior enhancement are predictive of benignity. This was the case in our study where the majority of the echogenic, homogeneous, well-limited image was present (83.3%).

The authors (39,54) considered that the anechoic image of well-defined shape, with clear, fine and regular limits with posterior enhancement typically proportional to the size and content of the cyst was consistent with fibrocystic dystrophy; this was found in our series.

Generally, large series (45) confirm the feasibility and diagnostic profitability of removal of breast lesions after ultrasound detection. **C- Malignant tumours :**

1- Correlation between mammography and histology :

The stellate form is the most classic form of breast cancer, it has been found in 56.2% of cancer cases, in the vast majority of cases it is an infiltrating ductal carcinoma more or less differentiated (45). Architectural disorganization is always indicative of a malignant pathology according to CHOPIER (28).

The higher proportion of microcalcifications representing 38% of the total radiological anomalies explored is found in other series (15).

The frequency of malignancy for each type of microcalcification compared to that of LAG is represented in the following table

Table 54: Comparative results according to LE GAL classification

Types	Le Gal (227)				Our study (42)			
	Total		Malin		Total		smart	
	Nb	%	Nb	%	Nb	%		
Type 1	11	5	2	5,5	0	0	0	0
Type 2	92	40	7	19,5	2	4,8	0	0
Type 3	40	18	4	14	5	11,9	4	9,5
Type 4	56	25	7	22	14	33,3	13	30,5
Type 5	28	12	16	44	21	50	21	50

This table confirms the definite benignity of type 1 microcalcifications and the malignancy

MCA type 5; which in all cases corresponded to cancer, on the other hand, a high frequency of malignancy was noted for MCA types 3 and 4.

According to the LE GAL model, the ACM foci are divided into 2 groups. Foci with more than 10 ACMs and their close groupings are significantly more frequent in cases of cancer (42.62%), in our series 50%. MILLIS found 72% of cancers for foci of more than 30 ACMs (24).

Thus, the triangular distribution of microcalcifications is found in 88% of carcinomas, as well as the polymorphic aspect within the same focus is present in 69% of cancers (24).

Five criteria are worth considering for the relative risk of increased breast cancer. These are: vermicular morphology of LE GAL type V, linear or branching description of the focus, number of calcifications >10/cm2, size of the focus >2 cm2 and irregularity in the size of the ACMs (24).

FRANCESHI notes that the association of MCA and opacity has the highest incidence of malignancy. Similarly, ROGERS finds 88% of cancers in lesions associating images with MCA foci (24). In our series this rate was 90.5%.

The correlation between mammographic appearance and malignant pathology is obtained in 91-96% in several studies. Fine analysis of mammographic lesions remains the most powerful predictor of cancer diagnosis (27, 31).

2- <u>Correlation between ultrasound and histology:</u>

Several ultrasound criteria deserve to be highlighted in malignant pathology:

- Heterogeneous, hypoechoic and irregular appearance of the images, found in 70% of the cancers (25) and 79.4% of the cancer cases in our study.

- Lack of well-defined shape, with interrupted wall on all sectional planes where the gap is visible (25).

- Long axis perpendicular to the skin is always very suspicious (24) as in our study where it was in 84.9% of cases.

- Attenuation of the posterior ultrasound beam is a classic sign, frequent (42.30% of cases) but not pathognomonic of cancer. If the diagnosis of malignancy is evoked on other criteria, posterior enhancement is not a criterion of exclusion; on the contrary (24).

DE MAULMONT reports in his study that the discovery of a tissue ultrasound nodule in contact with a focus of microcalcifications constitutes an argument in favour of the onset of invasion which could have escaped mammography (34).

Some difficulties in diagnosis are due to the ultrasound polymorphism of breast cancers which can have different appearances:

- a quasi-anechoic image: exceptional except for intramammary lymphomatous metastases (27).

- an isoechoic image: case of colloid cancers or cancers with sclerotic stroma, very calcified (37).

- a lacuna whose major axis is parallel to the skin: encountered in cases of lobular, medullary or colloid carcinoma (27).

However, it seems from the large series (54), that cysts are particularly well examined by ultrasound, and they are now less often subjected to cytopuncture. The existence of thick walls, irregular septa and endocystic vegetations have a better discriminatory value. Color Doppler ultrasonography finds its best indication here by authenticating tumor thickening and vascularization, and a lot of color signal in a tumor points to its malignant nature (24, 25).

VIGNAL (24) reports in his study that the sensitivity and specificity of ultrasound are respectively 88.9% and 97.9%.

If we compare the results of our series with those found in the literature we find :

- A study by COTTU (7) of 544 breast tumors reported that mammography and ultrasound had a sensitivity of 94% and specificity of 71%.

- Another study by CHOPIER (28) reported:

    S Of 62 benign tumours, 3 cases were mistaken for cancer (specificity: 95.2%).

    J Out of 64 cancers, the appearance was clearly malignant in 62 cases (sensitivity: 96.8%).

- In our series of 250 breast tumours, we found 84 benign tumours, i.e. 33.6%, and

146 malignant tumours, i.e. 58.4%, and 20 tumours of intermediate malignancy, i.e. 8%.

* of the 146 malignant tumours, 5 cases were mistaken for a benign aspect on mammography and 3 on ultrasound, i.e. :

* a mammographic sensitivity of 93.5%.

* and an ultrasound sensitivity of 93.8%.

* Of the 84 benign tumours, 16 cases were taken for breast cancer on mammography and 12 on ultrasound

Or :

* 86% mammographic specificity.

* and an ultrasound specificity of 89.7%.

If we compare the results of our series with those found in the literature, we find that our results are close to the other series with a sensitivity as high as the two series and a mammo-echographic specificity higher than that found in the series of COTTU, and less than that of the series of CHOPIER, we can thus conclude that mammography and ultrasound are sensitive but not very specific examinations for the evaluation of the type of breast tumors.

Anatomopathological examination remains the key examination, allowing the precise histological nature of breast tumours to be determined in order to evaluate the therapeutic attitude, the prognosis and the evolution.

D-HISTO RADIOLOGICAL COMPARISON ACCORDING TO THE ACR BIRADS CLASSIFICATION :

The BI-RADS™ lexicon is the first tool to standardize mammography reading and improve the accuracy of counts. It should help diagnose cancers at an early stage while avoiding unnecessary surgical biopsies (4, 7).

It includes 5 categories in which images are classified according to their degree of morphological suspicion, with an increasing positive predictive value of malignancy (17,18).

The classification of lesions into one of the categories 1 to 5, and especially into categories 3 to 5, is not always an easy task, even for an experienced senologist (19).

Some lesions appear quite benign but have discordant histologic findings, while many suspicious lesions are found to be benign on biopsy or surgery (17).

1-ACR2

Our study shows that the proportion of effectively benign lesions among images classified as ACR2 is 85.7% in mammography and 94.45% in ultrasound.

This rate is higher than 65 % and therefore satisfactory, as Wagon (17) points out Remember that the ACR2 classification implies the existence of a typically benign abnormality requiring neither special surveillance nor additional examination when the classification has been established.

2-ACR5 :

When an opacity was classified as ACR 5 in our study, the positive predictive value of the ACR 5 classification was good since 84 cancers were found on histology among the 86 lesions classified in this category on mammography, i.e., a malignancy rate of 97.6%, which is a very good figure when compared with other series that reported variable values in this category ranging from 54% (16) to 81% (17). These series were not limited to opacities and included cases of microcalcifications.

The malignancy rate in the series by Liberman et al. was 85% (17).

In the case of highly suspicious or multifocal ACR 5 lesions, biopsy allows optimization of therapeutic management.

Microbiopsy is then an effective alternative to surgical biopsy, replacing extemporaneous histological examination which is not recommended for lesions smaller than 1 cm (17).

Preoperative diagnosis will allow treatment in one anaesthetic step (immediate mastectomy or axillary curage in case of infiltrating lesion).

Some colleges, such as the European Society of Oncological Surgery (ESSO), recommend that more than 70% of cancers, whether palpable or not, be diagnosed cytologically or at best histologically before surgery (14). These practices also allow for accurate information to be given to the patient before considering therapeutic surgery, particularly in the case of mastectomy.

3-ACR4 :

The percentage of carcinoma for lesions classified as ACR 4 was 64.7% after surgical verification. This value is much better than that of the series of opacities by Liberman et al (17), which found a malignancy value of 35% for opacities in this category, and is consistent with the malignancy rate varying from 5 to 70% in this category according to ACR.

4-ACR3

Concerning lesions classified as ACR3; this category occurred with a frequency of 14.8% in our study, which is a high figure if we compare it to other series in the literature where it varied between 2% and 11%.

The proportion of actually benign lesions among these images was 78.9% in mammography and with an even better benignity rate in ultrasound of 86.5%.

The percentage of carcinoma for lesions classified as ACR 3 was 13.1% for mammography and 0% for ultrasound after definitive surgical verification, whereas the frequency of carcinoma for opacities in this category varies according to the series from 1.4% to 2% (15, 16), and is less than 5% according to the ACR

Therefore, this high figure compared to the other series and to the ACR classification is either due to an interpretation error having classified these lesions as ACR3 instead of ACR4, or indeed to an additional particularity of breast cancer in these 3 patients, one of whom had a history of breast cancer in her mother and another with a history of breast neo in her sister.

Consequently, it seems to us obligatory to biopsy lesions classified as ACR3 in patients with a particularly serious family or personal history; or to classify them as ACR4 since the classification takes risk factors into account.

5-Advantages and disadvantages of the ACR BI RADS classification :

1) Advantage:

In conclusion, we can say that our radiological interpretations appear encouraging since, among the 51 lesions diagnosed as benign by the radiologists (ACR2 and ACR3) in mammography, only 5 (9.8%) turned out to be malignant after definitive histological results, and among the 52 lesions classified ACR2 ACR3 in ultrasound, none (6%)

turned out to be malignant on histology.

Similarly, 75.8% of ACR4 lesions were actually malignant, thus justifying their biopsy. This rate is consistent with the ACR rate, which varies between 10 and 70% malignancy for ACR4.

Finally, it can be said that the PPV of benignity of ACR2 lesions and the PPV of malignancy of ACR5 are excellent. They therefore make it possible to avoid unnecessary lumpectomies for ACR2 which can be monitored over the long term and to reassure patients. They recommend extended surgery for RCC5 with clear carcinological objectives, i.e. obtaining satisfactory excision margins on histological study.

2) **disadvantages :**

This is especially problematic for ACR3 and ACR4 lesions, which remain difficult to interpret. The difference in classification between ACR3 and ACR4 can be complex. It is the clinical, family and personal history that will guide the senologist in his decision to biopsy the lesion or not. This is particularly the case for ACR3 for which we have found a higher rate of malignancy than that reported in the literature, which is normally less than 5% (17, 18, 19)

2.1. Problems encountered in the BI-RADS 4 and 5 categories

In some studies, readers may differ in their classification between categories 4 and 5 (18). However, in most cases this is of no practical consequence, as their recommendations for further investigations or biopsies are most often concordant (11). This concordance was 90-97% for cancers seen in screening and 91-96% for cancers detected by diagnostic mammography (12). Aspects with the highest PPV (spiculated contour, irregular shape, segmental or linear distribution) were classified as category 5 by the majority of authors. The highest PPV was for fine linear or tree-like calcifications and segmental distribution (13).

The diagnostic conclusions on lesions classified as ACR4 and 5 were correct in most cases in our study. For Bérubé et al the BIRADS ™ classification requires an ancillary method to reduce the number of lesions classified as category 4 or 5, found benign on biopsy results (19).

Ultrasound is very useful for opacities because it can confirm their solid nature. It also allows the diagnosis to be made more precisely by looking for criteria of benignity or malignancy (14), which are, however, subject to a certain interobserver variability (15). Unlike ultrasound, mammography cannot confirm or eliminate the existence of a mass. Some studies (16, 17, 18) have attempted to establish ultrasound criteria to distinguish between malignant and benign lesions with encouraging results, but most of the ultrasound characteristics are common to both benign and malignant tumours and it is the percutaneous biopsy that allows a conclusion to be reached.

In our series, the decision to perform a biopsy was made for lesions classified as Birads 4 or 5. The patient's clinical and radiological file was reviewed in a collegial manner, thus limiting the variability of mammographic interpretation between observers. All the radiological and clinical elements of each patient were taken into account before the biopsies were performed in order to optimize the management of the patients.

2.2. Problems encountered for category 3

When the lesions encountered are rigorously classified as BI-RADS 3, the various studies published show that the percentage of abnormalities classified in this category is moderate (2 to 11% of all lesions) and that the rate of cancer revealing itself during subsequent surveillance is very low (0.3 to 1.7%) (18). However, mammographic surveillance is sometimes erroneously recommended for lesions that retrospectively do not meet the diagnostic criteria for the BI-RADS 3 category (lesions/probably benign) (19)

The causes are: fatigue, inattention, lack of experience on the part of the reader; absence of the images necessary for correct diagnosis; a slowly growing tumour and absence of previous images for comparison; new masses or masses that have already increased in size; appearance of an intramammary pseudoganglion; consideration of the most reassuring criteria while ignoring the pejorative elements (19). To be classified as BI-RADS® 3, the lesion must be non-palpable, have undergone a complete diagnostic work-up and have been compared with previous examinations. For example, a slow-growing tumour may be diagnosed late and remain classified in category 3 for a longer or shorter period of time. Indeed, the perception of growth is sometimes delicate because it depends on the initial size of the lesion. The human eye perceives growth in diameter and not in volume. Small nodules appear to grow less rapidly than large ones, even if both double in volume at the same time. Thus a 5 mm nodule with a tumor doubling time of six months will see its diameter increase by only 1.25 mm. Conversely, changes in mammographic and/or ultrasound technique can modify the apparent diameter of an oval or lobulated nodule, leading to the belief that it is growing when in fact it is perfectly stable. There is still quite a lot of interobserver variation in the classification as category 3 or 4. Excessive BI-RADS 3 to BI- RADS 4 classification reduces the specificity of guided and surgical biopsies and increases the number of unnecessary invasive procedures (19). This risk exists all the more so because to cover himself from a possible medicolegal recourse, the radiologist may be tempted to upgrade to BI-RADS 4 in order to have a biopsy performed at the slightest doubt. However, this risk is fairly small because the BI-RADS classification, which is American in conception, includes this parameter and already allows a very wide latitude in the indication for biopsies. On the other hand, a reader with an abnormally high rate of BIRADS 3 lesions will probably allow a certain number of proven cancers to develop, the prognosis of which could be altered if the patient's compliance with short and medium term surveillance is not good (19).

Therefore, in conclusion, if we take into account the results of our series, and given the high rate of malignancy in this category, lesions classified as ACR3 must necessarily benefit from close surveillance, and may in the case of a serious personal or family history be reclassified as ACR4.

VIII-Interest of the clinical-radiological-histological association :

In total, the diagnostic concordance of the 3 means of senological diagnosis was found in 230 cases. Concordance of the diagnosis with the histological results was found in 206 cases, i.e. 89.6% of cases.

Comparison of these results with those obtained for each element of the diagnosis separately shows that this combination provides better results with greater accuracy and fewer false diagnoses.

Indeed, if a single element of this association affirms malignancy, the value of the diagnostic method that shows this malignancy must be taken into account and confirmed by an extemporaneous biopsy.

In conclusion, it can be said that this association remains very relevant in the diagnosis of breast cancer.

Conclusion

Diagnosing breast disease is a difficult art, even for a trained team,

For the moment, our brains and our eyes are still much more efficient, provided that we train them with competent people, constantly question ourselves and follow a rigorous approach using all the means at our disposal to arrive at a diagnosis. Today, we can reasonably propose:

The results of our series confirm the importance of the clinical examination in the diagnosis of breast tumours

This classification uses a standardized description to refine the results for both mammography and ultrasound, and leads to recommendations for clinical practice.

Mammography, being the key diagnostic examination and the first radiological examination that has been able to reproduce the mammary gland and its abnormalities on X-rays, still retains its place in breast pathology and is tending towards perfection, always in association with ultrasound, which is an integral part of all breast exploration and which provides important information where mammography is less effective, particularly in the exploration of dense breasts, as our study shows. Indeed, pathological analysis of the radiological aspect obtained seems to allow a better diagnostic approach with a histological concordance of 86 to 94%.

The search for an optimal sensitivity/specificity ratio requires radiological quality control and consensual decision-making by the surgeon, radiologist and pathologist.

The third interest is the practice of percutaneous tissue sampling, the indication of which is to be discussed in a multidisciplinary manner. Micro and macro biopsies remain an important link in the chain, but it is better to train and set up a close and real collaboration between the radiologist, the pathologist and the surgeon with a permanent confrontation of our results.

Anatomopathological examination remains the fundamental examination to determine the benign or malignant nature of the tumour.

SUMMARY

Breast pathology occupies a very important place among women's pathologies and still constitutes a problem for practitioners in terms of both diagnosis and treatment.

Clinical, mammography and ultrasound are the main methods of breast diagnosis, hence the need to verify the respective values of each method by comparing them with the final histological results.

Our work based on the study of 250 cases of breast tumors, collected in the department of obstetrics and gynecology II of the CHU HASSAN II of Fez, during 2 years between 2011 and 2012 has allowed us to highlight the following points: - Breast pathology seems to affect the female population at any age with a peak frequency between 36 and 45 years.

• The breast nodule is the revealing symptom of breast tumors in 96.8% of cases.

• The superolateral quadrant is the most frequent location of breast tumors in 36% of cases.

• Malignant tumours (58.4%) are slightly more frequent than benign tumours (33.6%).

• Invasive ductal carcinoma predominated (49.6%), as did histopronostic grade SBR II-III.

• The clinical examination, the first indispensable diagnostic step, has a diagnostic sensitivity of 97.03%.

• Mammography was sensitive in 93.8% of cases and specific in 89.7% of cases. - Breast ultrasound is sensitive in 93.5% of cases, and specific in 86% of cases.

• The PPV of benignity of lesions classified as ACR2 (98.8%), and the PPV of malignancy of lesions classified as ACR5 (94%) are excellent.

• The malignancy rate is high in the ACR3 category (13.1%)

The results of the clinical-radiological-histological association are much better than those obtained for each separate means of diagnosis, with a histological concordance of 100% for malignant tumours and 97.67% for benign tumours, i.e. 98.97% of cases for all benign and malignant tumours.

References:

1 . Association lalla salma of fight against the breast cancer
2 . Epidemiology of breast cancer in Morocco (INO patients between 1985-2002)
3 . JEAN PHILIPPE BERETTES, CAROLE MATHELIN , BEATRICE GAIRARD , JEAN PIERRE BELLOCQ Livre cancer du sein Masson ed 2007
4 . FARKI M medical thesis casa 199 n°229
5 . MATHELIN. C Clinical examination of breast cancer. Encycl. Méd. Chir 1997, 865-C-10 : 10p
6 . ROUESSE. J Malignant tumours of the breast. Rev. Pratique. Gynécol. Obstét 1995, 45.
7 . COTTU.P.H Retrospective multivariate analysis of the radio-anatomical-pathological correlation of subclinical breast lesions. Rev. Internal Medicine 2000, 21: 337-343.
8 . J WANG, LL FAJARDO, L DAHMOUCH , MW VANNIER . Lobular carcinoma in situ presenting as architectural distortion on mammography: a case report and review of the literature. European journal of Radiology extra 2004; 50:63-66
9 . PARK JM, HAN BK, MOON WK, CHOE YH, AHN SH, GONG G. Metaplastic carcinoma of the breast: Mammographic and sonographic findings. J ClinUltrasound 2000;28:179-86. magerie de la Femme, Volume 18, Issue 4, December 2008, Pages 247-250
10 PHILIPPA.M. L Correlation between ultrasound characteristics, mammographic findings and histological grade in patients with invasive ductal carcinoma of the breast. Clinical Radiology 2000, 55: 40-44.
11 LANSAC. J Pathology of the breast. Gynaecology for the practitioner, Ed. 1994.
12 EL GHAOUI.A Breast cancers revealed by microcalcifications without palpable tumor. Rev. Fr. Gynécol. Obstét 1998, 93, 5: 361-369.
13 HALL.N.J Bilateral breast carcinomas: do they have similar mammographic features? Clinical Radiology 1999, 54: 434-437.
14 .SG OREL, N KAY , C REYNOLDS, DC SULLIVAN . BIRADS categorisation as a predictor of malignancy . Radiology 1999 .211(3) :845-850
15 .KOPANS DB, Mammography screening for breast cancer . cancer 1993,72,1809
16 .M EPSIE, A DE ROQUANCOURT , B TOURNANT , F PERRET . Benign masthopathy and risk of breast cancer. Advanced techniques in gynecology.
17 GARNIER.C Fibroadenoma of the breast: correlation between histology and dynamic MRI Medical thesis. Paris, 1995, n°95PA060055.
18 VESELY. M Distinction of phyllode tumor from fibroadenoma. Cancers 2000, 90, 6.
19 LE TREUT. Benign masthopaties.Arnette Blackwell, Ed. 1995
20 .DENT DM, CANT PJ. Fibroadenoma. World J Surg 1989;13:706-10.
21 MATAR. N Phyllodes tumors of the breast. Rev. Fr. Gynécol. Obstét 1998, 93, 5: 335-339

22 .JABOT, E GRARDEL-CHANI BENOIT, F AUQUIER , C RENARD , A BRUNIAU , PLEHMANN and A RENOND journal of radiology vol 89 ; issue 10 at 2008

23 CHAOS TC , LOYF , CHEN SC , CHEN MF senografic features of phyllodes tumors of the breast ultrasound obtetrics and gynecology 2002 ;20 :64- 71

24 FLEURY, P Breast microcalcifications. Imagerie du sein JFR 1996, 4760.

25 .WA BERG, CI CAMPASSI , OB IOFFE , cystic lesions of the breast : stenographic pathologic correlations . Radiology 2003 ; 227 :183-191

26 .HARVE MIGNOTTE, book : Breast diseases Masson ed 2011-07-02

27 KECHAOU, H. DERBALI, S. OUESLATI, A. AYEDI, H. BOUBAKER, E. SFAR, M. CHAABANE, Inflammatory pathology with clinical, mammographic and ultrasound variable expression sometimes suspicious Journal de Radiologie, Volume 90, Issue 10, October 2009, Page1610 S.

28 .J. CHOPIER, N. KADIA, S. GUILBOT, C. SALEM AND C. Marsault Paris - La pathologie inflammatoire subaigue ou chronique mammaire ,France Journal de Radiologie, Volume 85, Issue 9, September2004, Page 1250 J. Chopier, N. Kadi, S. Guilbot, C. Salem, C. Marsault

29 .S GREENSTEIN OREL, CS DOUGHERTY, C Reynolds, BJ CZERNIECKI , ES SIEGELMAN , MD SCHNALL . MR imaging in patients with nipple discharge: initial experience . Radiology 2000; 215:248-254

30 R. GUILLIN, S. TAIEB, L. DESCHILDRE, H. BERCE, F. BACHELLE, C. CHAVERON, L. CEUGNART cytosteatonecrosis typical and atypical aspects journal of Radiology, Volume 87, Issue 10, October 2006, Page 1554

31 SYLVIA H, HEYWANG KOBRUNNER, INGRID SCHREER Imagerie diagnostique du sein Masson ed 2007 ; pages 19-96

32 JAQUES SAGLIER , PHYLIPPE BEUZEBO , ARLETTE POMMEYRO Masson ed 2009

33 .NETTER. E et al. Ductal carcinoma in situ of the breast: place of imaging. Journal Radiol 1998, 79: 651-658.

34 .DE MAULMANT.C Forty years of progress in breast imaging. Pathol. Biol 2000, 48 : 801-811.

35 KYUNG-SANG. L Correlation between mammographic manifestations and averaged histopathologic nuclear grade using prognosis-predict scoring system for the prognosis of ductal carcinoma in situ. Clinical Imaging 1999, 23: 339-346.

36 POPLAK AND WELLS Ductal carcinoma in situ of the breast: mammographic-pathologic correlation. AJR 1998, 170: 1543-1549.

37 CARLSON.K.L Relationship between mammographic screening intervals and size and histology of ductal carcinoma in situ. AJR 1999, 172 : 313317.

38 GIRAUD.PH, CASELLES.O ET AL Detection of foci of microcalcifications, contribution of the digital image. J. Le sein 1996, 6, 1 : 10-18.

39 GEORGIAN-SMITH.D Calcifications of lobular carcinoma in situ of the breast: radiologic-pathologic correlation. AJR 2001, 176: 1255-1259.

40 TOUBOUL. E Preoperative dose chemotherapy and radiotherapy of locally

advanced, non-inflammatory breast cancers of more than 3 cm in diameter. Sem. Hôp. Paris 1997, 73: 23-24.

41 TOIKKA.NENS. Primary squamous cell carcinoma of the breast. Cancer 1981, 48: 1629-32.

42 BOGOMOLETZ W.V., Pure squamous cell carcinoma of the breast. Arch. Path. Lab Med. 1982, 106: 57 -9

43 SHOUSHAS JAMES A.H., FERNANDEZ M.D., BULL T.B. Squamous cell carcinoma Of the breast. Arch. Path. Lab. Med 1984, 108: 893-6.

44 .JINY. CAMPANA F. VILLOQJ. R et al. Primary squamous cell carcinoma of the breast Clinical, histopathological and prognostic study of 14 patients. Bull. Cancer 1992, 79: 675-9.

45 .E RUBIN, D VISCHER, R ALEXANDER , M URIST. Proliferative disease and atypia in biopsies performed for nonpalpable lesions detected mammographycally , Cancer 1988 ; 61 :2077-2082.

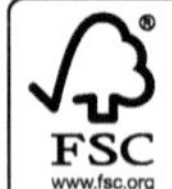

Printed by Books on Demand GmbH, Norderstedt / Germany